Natural Ceramics

David Korson
Dental Technician
London, England

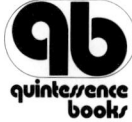

Quintessence Publishing Co. Ltd. 1990
Chicago, London, Berlin, Tokyo, São Paulo

British Library Cataloguing in Publication Data
Korson, David
  Natural ceramics.
  1. Prosthetic dentistry
  I. Title
  617.69

  ISBN 1-85097-015-7

Typesetting, printing and binding: Kösel, Kempten, West-Germany
Lithography: Toppan Printing Co. (S) Pte. Ltd., Singapore
Printed in West-Germany

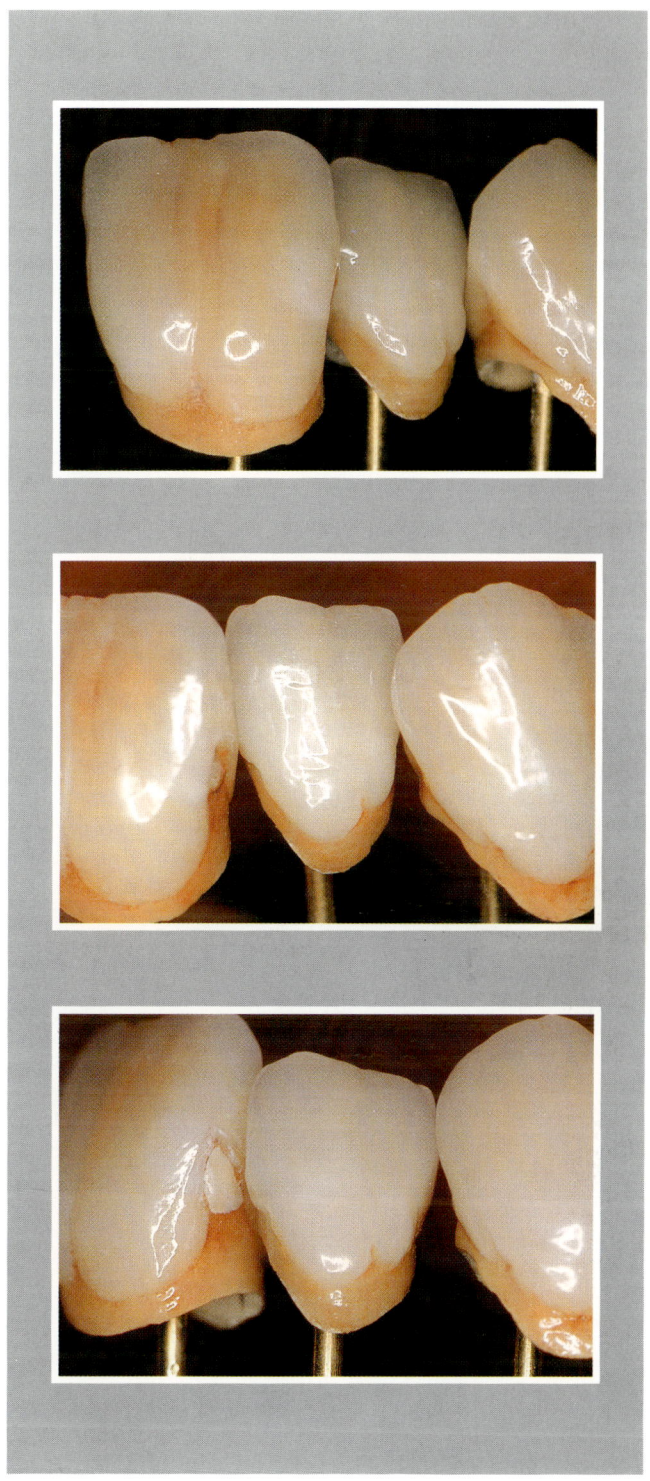

Figs A to C
Anterior Jacket Crowns for the aged dentition.
Building ceramics with character in order to duplicate natural dentition is a rewarding challenge. Chapters relating the principles and techniques will explain in detail the way to achieve this.

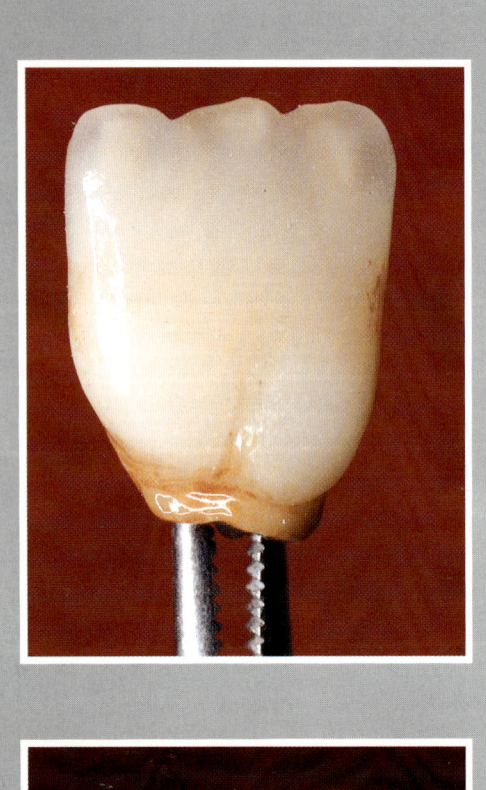
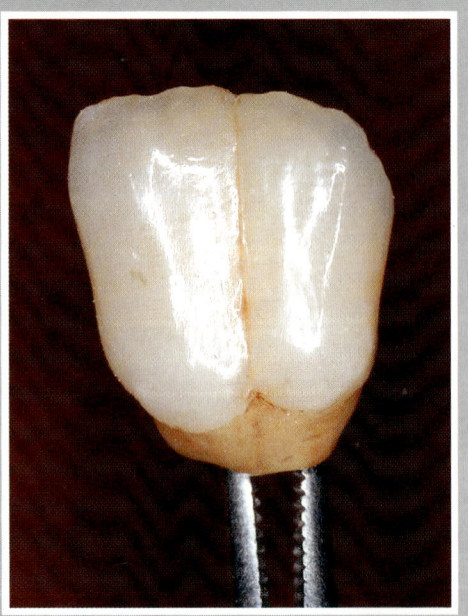
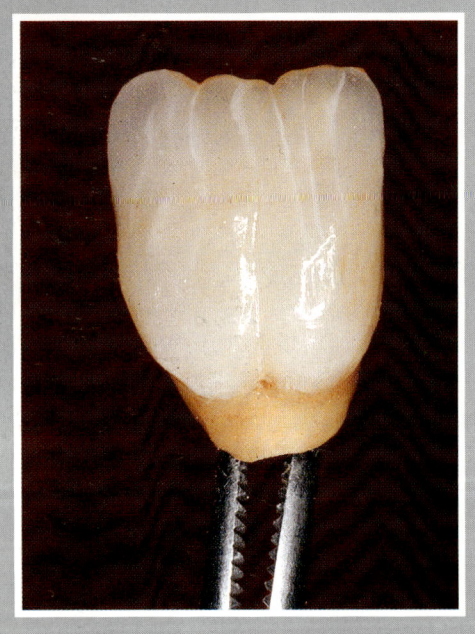
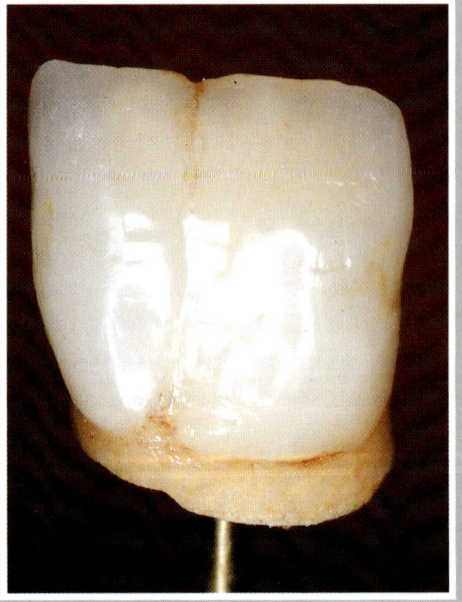

Figs D to G (page 6)
Individuality – nature as demonstrated in four anterior restorations.
The Visual Building Technique detailed within this book will explain many possibilities for duplicating natural effects which make human dentition so individual.

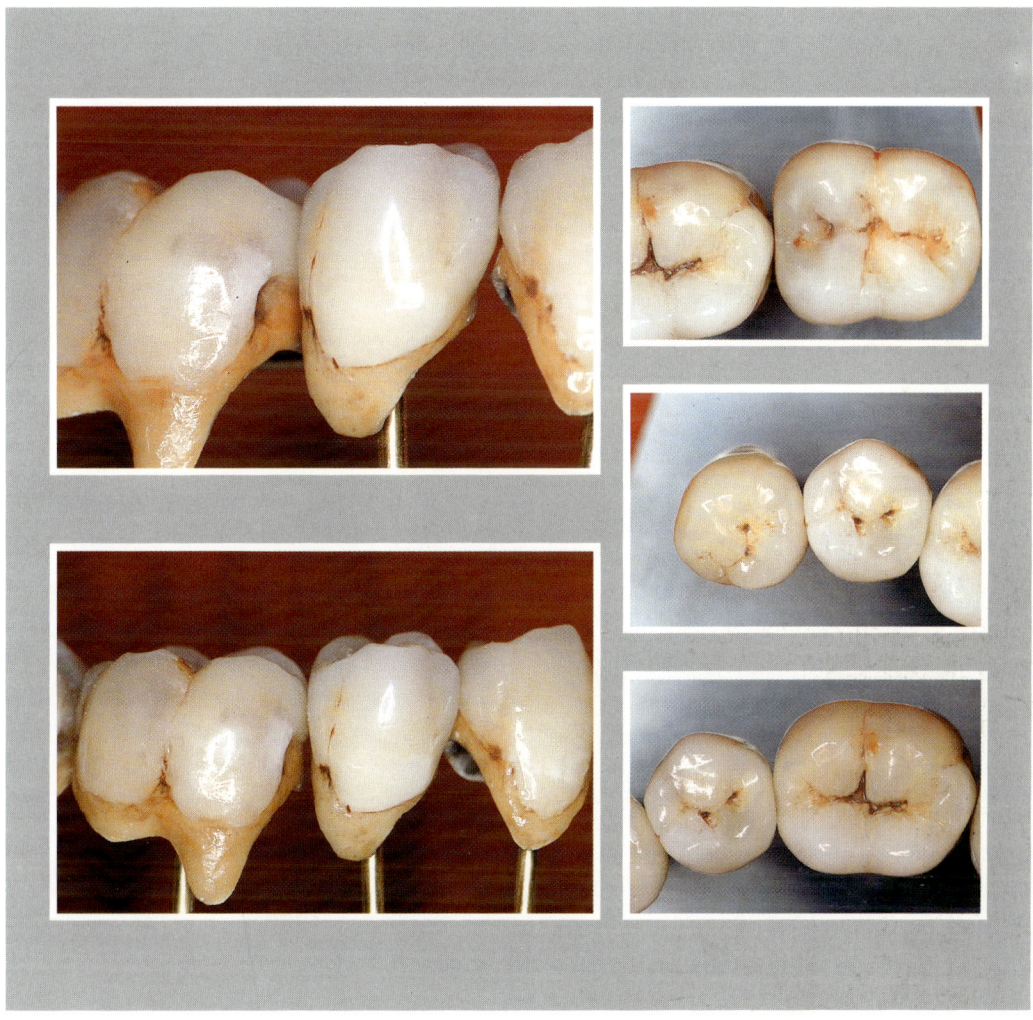

Figs H to L (above)
Characteristics of Posterior Dentition.
Metal ceramic examples.

Foreword

To many patients who require anterior ceramic reconstruction, the prime importance will be aesthetics and for the dental ceramist to achieve this, close involvement with the patient is necessary. The selection of porcelain colours to exactly match natural dentition in position, depth and intensity, requires precise shade selection technique and the necessary skill and expertise to create in porcelain the reality of an artificial tooth which will be undetectable to visual inspection.

The successful restoration will, of course, depend upon surgical procedures and close co-operation between dentist and technician in many areas, not least the critical area of tooth reduction and the preparation for the crown margin.

Tooth morphology is of particular importance for the biological acceptability of the restoration, as incorrect axial wall profile or occlusal disharmony may have catastrophic effect upon the tissues, musculature and remaining dentition.

The extent of knowledge and artistic ability bears a direct relationship to the accomplishment of the aesthetic and functional ideal, therefore both must be developed.

Finally a passion for achieving the highest possible standard in everything will result in eventual success.

Acknowledgements

Compiling this book has taken many hours of labour and I could not have written it without the help and encouragement of my wife *Valerie*, whose painstaking interpretation of my ideas into graphic illustrations has improved the work immeasurably, in addition her preparation of the manuscript took a great deal of time and patience. For all this and her encouragement and forbearance during those bleak times when things did not go to plan, my love and appreciation.

I would also like to thank both Mr *H. W. Haase* and Mr *John Brooks* for their encouragement and support.

Finally my thanks must go to Dr *John McLean* not only for reading and commenting on the script but also for the inspiration he has given to myself and to many others involved in dental ceramics.

Preface

Metal ceramics still remain the most widely-used materials in fixed prosthodontics, and advances in the formulation and technology of the veneer porcelains during the last two decades have transformed our concepts of what can be achieved in aesthetic dentistry. *David Korson* has pioneered the development of high chroma dentines and this book illustrates the remarkable strides that he has made in overcoming the problem of duplicating natural root effects. No longer is it necessary to use surface staining to mask unsightly gingival opaque porcelains which plagued the dental ceramist for so long. This book also gives the reader an insight into *David Korson's* thorough understanding of tooth anatomy which he conveys with clear diagrams and colour illustrations. Layering and segmental building of the enamel veneers has been a strong feature in *David's* work and resulted in his gaining the first Fellowship of the International Society for Dental Ceramics for his ceramic demonstration case.

The beginner will gain inspiration from this book and the advanced ceramist may also find areas where he still can make further improvements. *David Korson* was the first Editor of the International Society for Dental Ceramics magazine "Excellence" and this book truly shows his pursuit of this elusive goal.

Dr *John W. McLean*, OBE FDS RCS (Eng) DSc MDS (Lond) Dr Odont (Lund)
Consulting Professor in Fixed Prosthodontics and Biomaterials, Louisiana State University

Contents

1 Tooth Character in the Maxilla

Anterior aesthetics are of prime importance to many individuals. Multiple restorations require artistry and a sympathetic understanding of the needs of the patient. Tooth size, shape and position affect the overall appearance in extensive restoration of anterior teeth. Age and sex can be an important factor in establishing facial aesthetics.

Therefore this chapter details the character and individuality of each anterior tooth in the maxilla, and their effect as a group. The special needs of the older female who wishes to recapture youthful beauty are considered as this is a common situation, with which we all have to deal.

1.1 Natural Character of Teeth

A prerequisite to fabricating aesthetically pleasing artificial teeth must be an understanding of tooth position and the way slight alterations to inclination – particularly in anterior teeth – can influence the overall functional and aesthetic effect. The importance each tooth has to the arrangement, the contribution careful shade selection can make in creating a natural appearance and the break-up of colour both from tooth to tooth and within each tooth is essential.

Centrals

The face and lips play an important role in the sensuality of an attractive woman; when the lips part the dominance of the upper centrals is of vital importance to the smile. In many cases this is achieved by lengthening or making in a lighter colour. Large centrals often create an attractive appearance (fig 1).

As the dentition ages, dominance of the centrals lessens to some degree and sexuality ceases to be a factor. However, when patients observe their teeth it is those in the front which are first seen and most critically assessed, particularly if they are part of a restoration. In an extensive rehabilitation these teeth play an important role and acceptance will influence the judgement of the complete aesthetic appeal.

Laterals

Laterals should be dainty and in harmony with the centrals, enhancing the character of the smile whilst being less prominent. A slight twist in the axis of the tooth prevents an artificial appearance.

Incisal edge profile is important and in the young female a rounded incisal edge aids femineity. As the dentition ages the incisal edges will become worn flat through attrition.

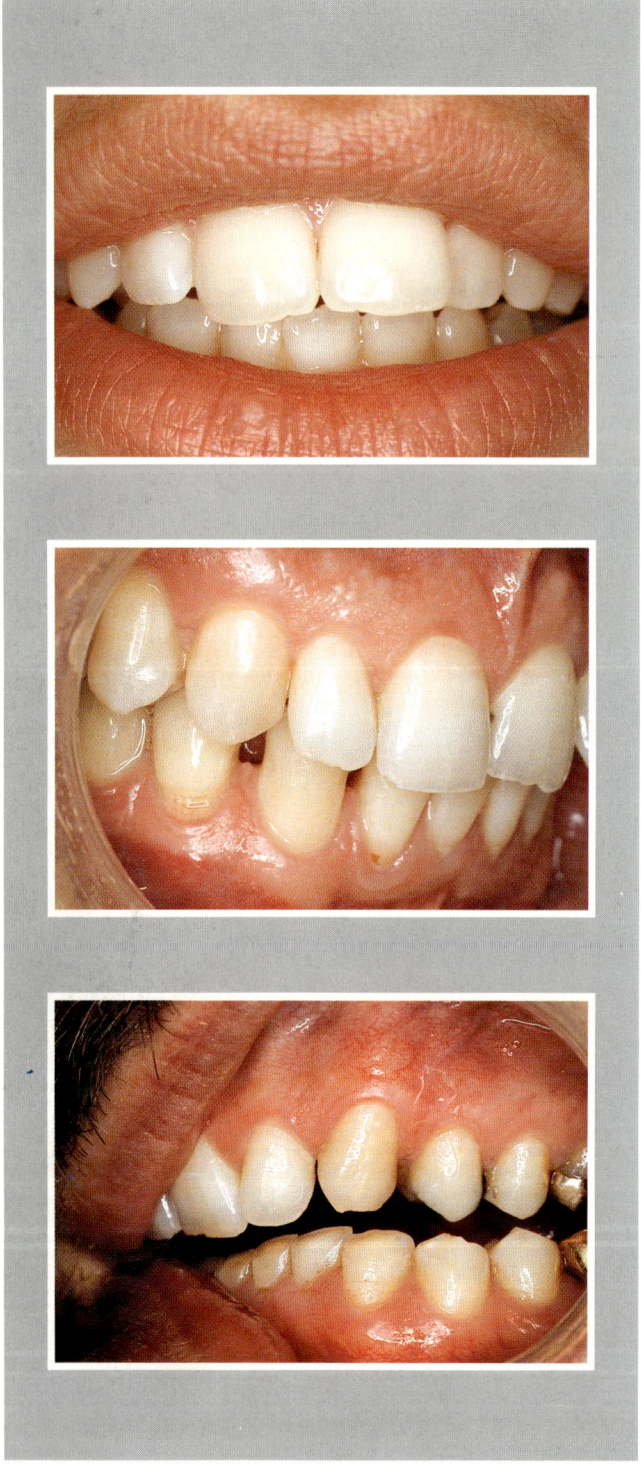

Fig 1 Large centrals create a sensual appearance in the young female.

Fig 2 Dainty lateral and pointed teeth create a youthful appearance.

Fig 3 Canine worn flat by attrition giving an aged appearance.

Figs 4 and 5 Examples of mono-chromatic shading in existing restoration and of suggested colour combination in new crowns.

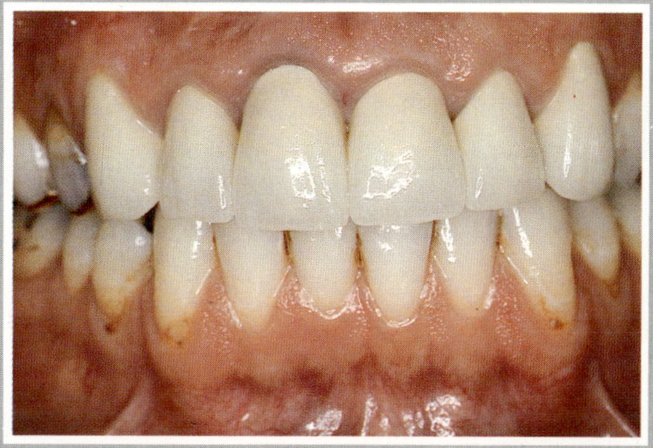

Fig 4 The patient intended to replace this restoration due to the monochromatic nature of the teeth and lack of individuality from tooth to tooth.

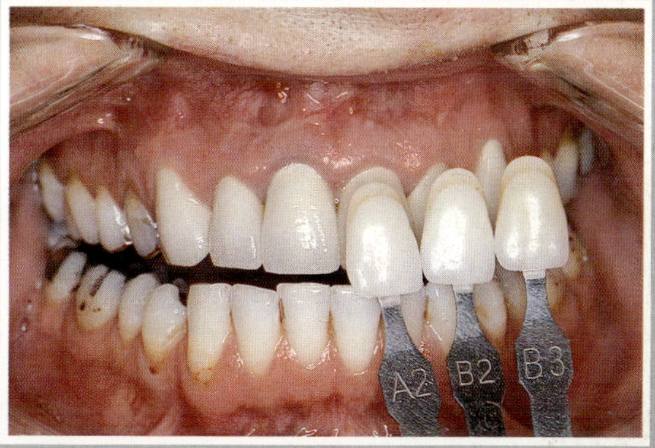

Fig 5 Patient aged 25 wished to have light coloured teeth. The colour combination chosen was Vita A2 centrals, subdued laterals B2 and darker canine teeth B3.

Canines

The corner stone of the dental arch, this tooth must dominate its neighbours without detracting from the importance of the centrals.

The young tooth has a cuspid tip shape. A youthful appearance will be enhanced by creating a dainty pointed cusp. With age the cusp tip will become flattened by abrasion (figs 2 and 3).

With multiple restorations aesthetic advantage can result from varying the shades between teeth. Almost always the canines should be at least one shade darker and the laterals slightly lower in value, thereby increasing the value of the centrals. In the younger patient, the youthful middle-aged and for those wishing whitish teeth, the centrals are created lighter than the laterals. In the older patient dominance may be achieved by the use of darker centrals (figs 4 and 5).

Table 1 Suggested colour combinations for patients who require complete anterior restoration.

	Centrals	Laterals	Canines
For a young person	B1	A1	A2
	A1	A1	A2
	B2	A2	A3
	A2	B2	B3
For the middle-aged person	D2	C1	D3
	B2	D3	A3.5
	A2/C1/C2	D3	B3
For an older person	B4	B3	A4
	B4	C3	C4
	A3.5	A4	C4
	C3	C2	C4

1.2 The Hollywood Smile

We have all experienced the middle-aged lady who requests "white teeth", accepting nothing darker than Vita A1. This patient wishes to have perfect teeth similar to the young models seen on magazine covers. The illusion of perfect teeth is caused by their framed appearance between parted lips, contrasting white against a vermillion background. In the young female this appearance is exaggerated by lipstick.

Treatment requires understanding. We must not forget that our patient has probably lived for many years with chipped and discoloured teeth which are ugly in appearance, so that showing teeth by laughing and even smiling has become something to avoid. It is in this situation that teeth become a phobia and other peoples' teeth become the envy of our patient. Given the opportunity to renew their appearance it is not surprising that so many strongly request clean white teeth with an even arrangement, in an effort to correct all the faults in the original teeth.

Fabricating a row of monochromatic white teeth of even size and uniform distribution will result not in youthful and perfect teeth but in a bright artificial denture-like appearance.

Careful explanation to the patient, with the aid of photographs from magazines and dental photographs of young perfect teeth should educate the patient to a more enlightened understanding of what teeth really look like. Whilst a light shade may still be chosen, the ceramist will be able to create a natural and pleasing aesthetic appearance (figs 6 to 8).

Figs 6 to 8 Case Study.
Middle aged female patient requested even arrangement and white colour for the restoration of her maxillary anterior teeth. After patient education an understanding was reached, expectations were altered slightly towards a more realistic approach.

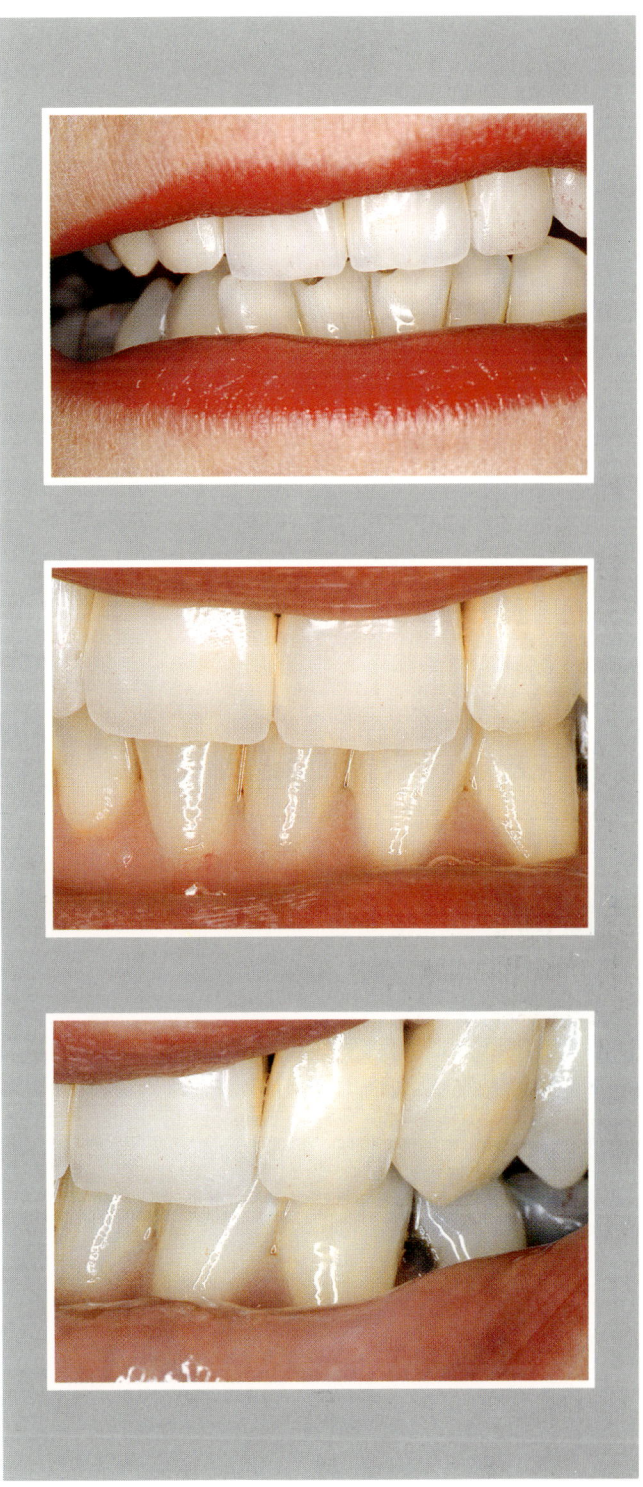

Fig 6 13 to 23 were fabricated moderately even. Subtle tooth position, shape and internal colour blending combine to create an aesthetic result.

Fig 7 Close detail photograph demonstrates realistic ceramic surfaces and harmonious blending with lower incisors.

Fig 8 Lateral view. Central is built in shade Vita A2 to create a light appearance. Lateral in A3 to blend the canine which is A3.5. The result is a harmonious arrangement with the lower incisors and maxillary posterior teeth. The patient's expectations were fulfilled (surgeon *Alodia Wojcik*).

2 The Art of Matching Teeth to People

Lighting conditions can have an effect on our perception of basic colour distribution; good lighting is a prerequisite for accurate colour assessment.

The task of the dental ceramist is to build a restoration to suit the individual. High standards of aesthetics can only be accomplished by the ceramist meeting the patient several times, which requires a degree of willingness and co-operation by both dentist and patient.

In this chapter procedures for shade selection and final corrections are discussed.

2.1 Lighting Conditions

Many problems occur during the initial matching procedure especially with regard to proper lighting conditions. These are essential for correctly determining the degree and translucency of the enamel overlay and the intensity and hue of mamelons and other incisal effects.

Establishing the best environment to view teeth has and still does present many problems. Due to the nature of crowns with thin sections and the various layers of porcelain, problems of metamerism often arise. It is impossible to achieve a result that will appear in the same way as natural dentition under all lighting conditions, but both natural daylight from a large window and an artificial light source should be available.

The colours we observe are dependent upon the quality of the light available for viewing. They vary according to their wavelength and to extraneous reflections from coloured walls, clothing etc. as well as with the intensity of light.

A balanced spectrum of light is essential, as an incorrect light source will create a bias in our perception towards the colour of the illuminants.

A tungsten filament light has a low colour temperature and is in the yellow colour range. This will effect the colour we perceive, as light waves in the blue range will not be present and therefore cannot transmit these hues back to the observer. The tungsten filament bulb will have a colour bias which will alter what may be a Vita D2 to appear more yellow, similar to Vita A2.

Conversely a colour selection taken early in the morning when there is a blue sky will have a dominant blue bias from the reflection and could alter Vita A2 to appear as Vita D2 (figs 9 and 10).

The correct colour determination for such characteristics as mamelons, incisal translucent areas and halo effects as well as for areas of opalescence in enamel requires the best possible conditions for viewing (figs 11 and 12).

As natural daylight contains the most balanced colour spectrum, it is the ideal light

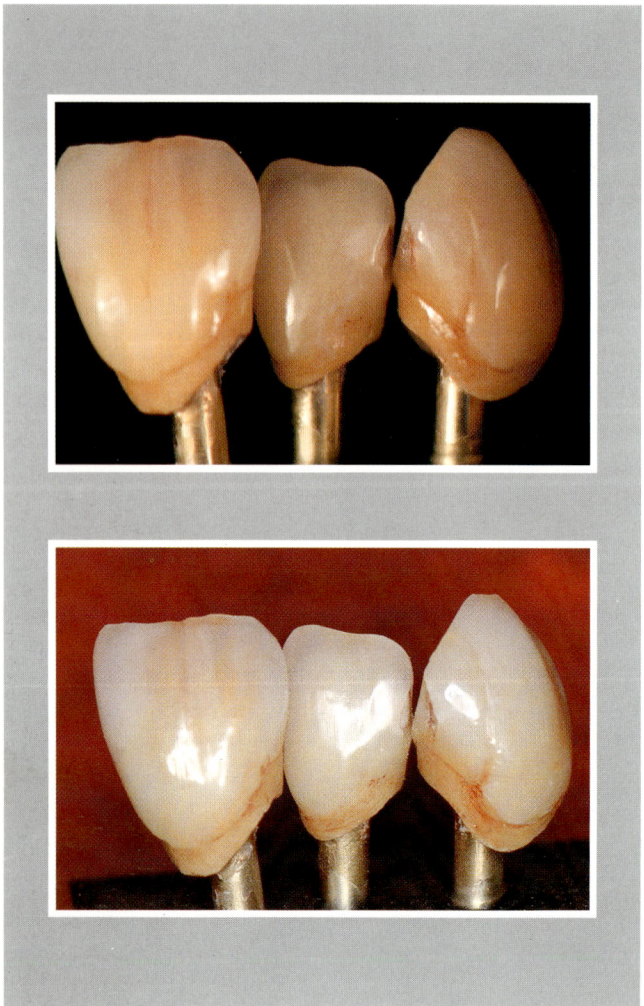

Figs 9 and 10 Photographs taken under different lighting conditions demonstrate mismatching. The importance of correct lighting for shade selection procedures cannot be over stressed if this and similar problems are to be avoided.

Fig 9 Demonstrates the effect when a tungsten filament lamp is used. The low kelvin temperature and strong yellow bias produces a dark yellow tint.

Fig 10 Correct colour of phantom case.

source to take shades as in this way fewer problems will emerge when observing the resultant ceramic under differing light sources. Even so, natural light is not ideal at all times, due to the way in which the sunlight scatters as it travels through the atmosphere[1]. During early morning and evening there is a predominant red bias; on a sunny day with little cloud a strong blue bias influences our judgement. Only in mid-morning and mid-afternoon when there is light cloud scattering to defuse an otherwise

Table 2 depicts the colour temperature of familiar light sources.

Tungsten filament bulb	2,500k
Photo floodlight	3,200–3,400k
Fluorescent Tubes range	4,000–6,000k
Daylight early morning	2,000k
mid-morning	5,500k
mid-day	up to 10,000k
mid-afternoon	5,500k
evening	2,000k

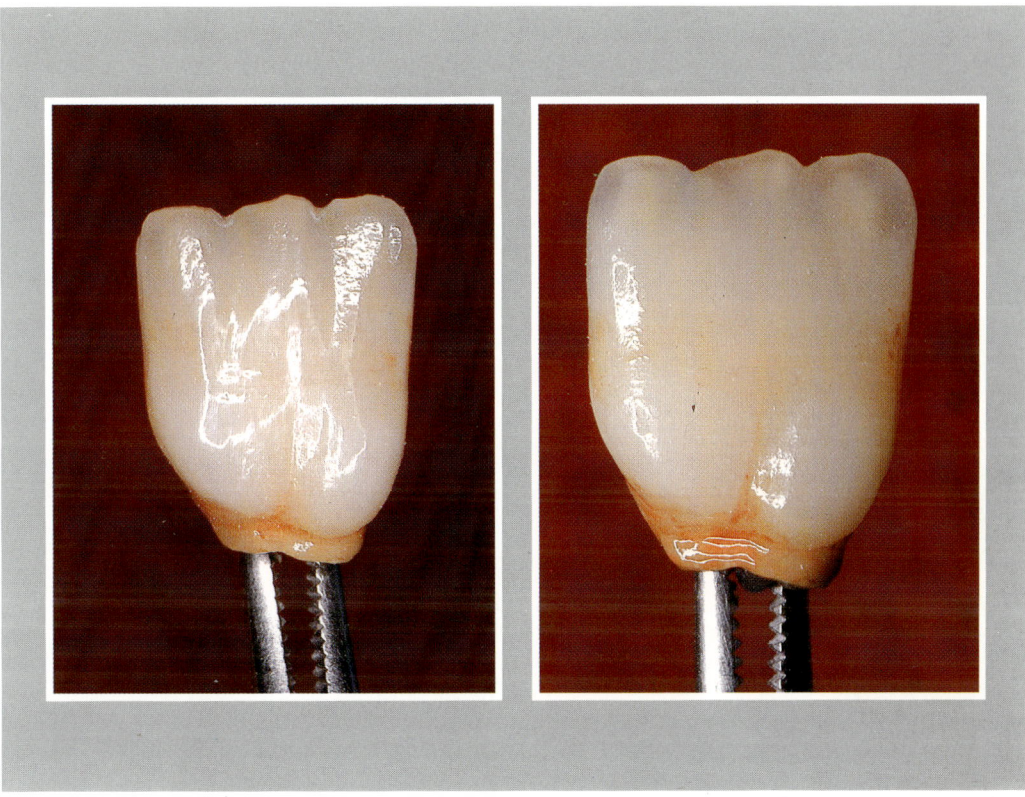

Figs 11 and 12   High reflection and too much light have created a situation where the subtle nuances of character within the crown are hidden. Translucency, mamelons and depth have all been lost (right). The many different colour characteristics within teeth are more easily observed when differing light sources are used.

blue sky are there ideal conditions for shade selection.[2, 3]

Whilst daylight conditions may be ideal at certain times of the day, this is not suitable for working practice or consistent results.

Although not as accurate as ideal daylight, fluorescent tubes for colour matching* are available and may be mounted in standard fittings. Dental surgery and laboratory lighting should be of this description.

Application

It is preferable for the shade selection pro-

cedures to be taken with the patient in either a sitting or standing position with their teeth in a horizontal plane to the observer's eye. Ceiling-mounted fluorescent tubes place the dentition in shadow in this position and therefore a portable light which can be positioned in front of the patient is required.

Artificially-created full-spectrum illuminants specifically designed for shade selection in dentistry are available (Waldmann** Color-i-Dent II) and these offer an alternative light source in which to view teeth. Because of the constant conditions these are more reliable than daylight.

* Color Rite. Thorn EMI plc London, England True-Lite, Duro Test Corporation, North Bergen, NJ 07047, USA.

** Waldmann, D-7730 Villingen-Schwenningen, W. Germany.

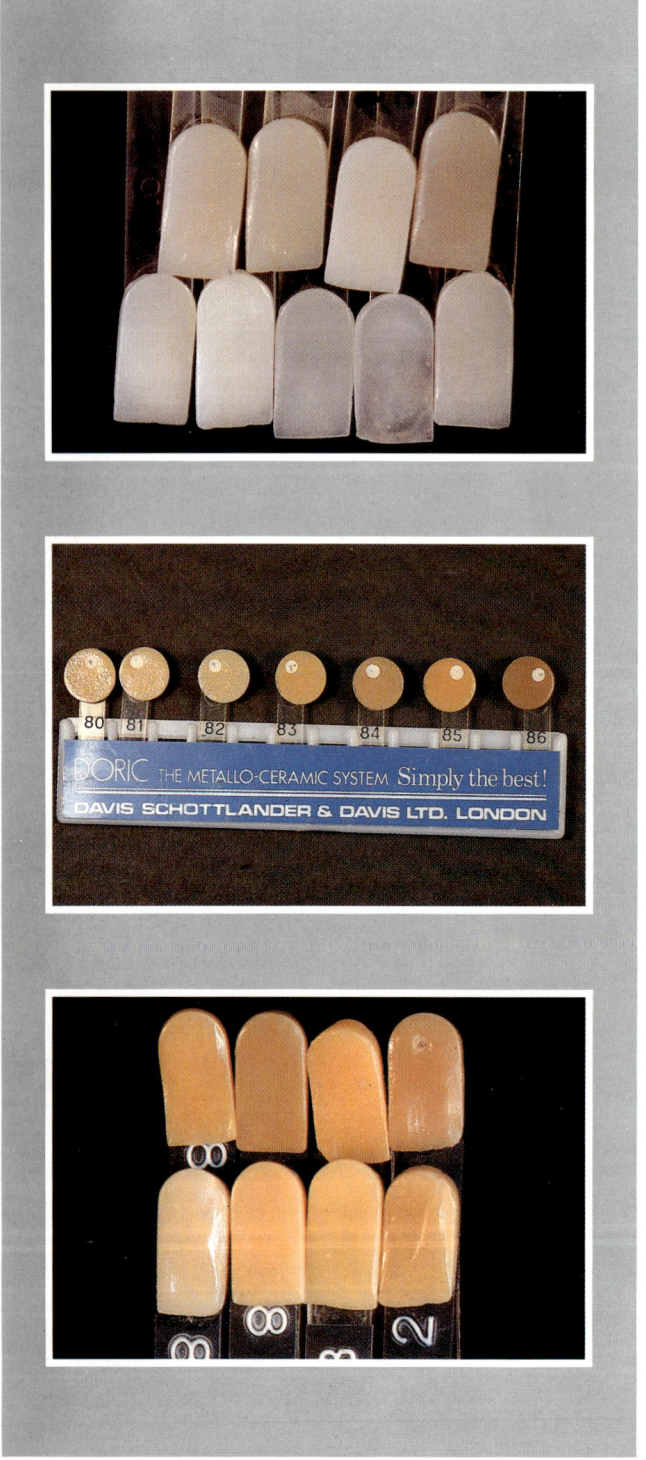

Fig 13 Enamel guides are used to check enamel overlays during shade selection and as an indication of value, opacity and translucency during building.

Figs 14 and 15 High Chroma Dentines formulated both in Doric and in Vita porcelain are used to evaluate areas where dentine has become exposed through either abrasion or tissue recession.

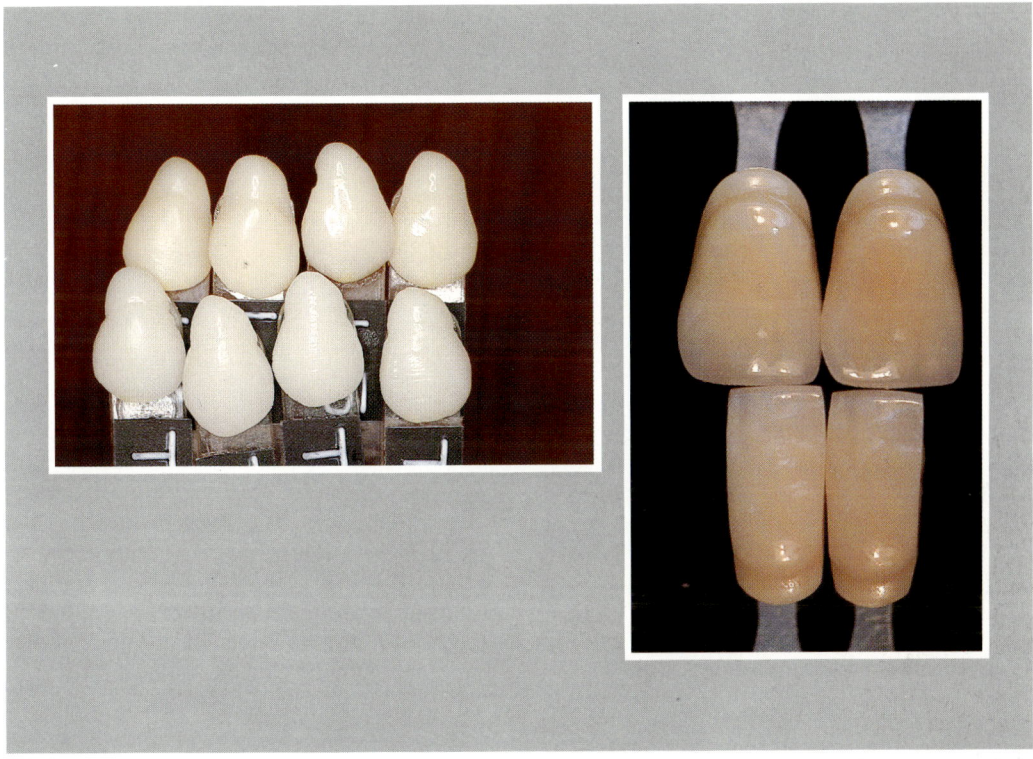

Fig 16 (left)   Texture and lustre guides help to provide useful communication between dentist and technician when they are apart and the technician is unable to see the patient.

Fig 17 (right)   In many cases uncertainty exists during shade selection between two hues on the commercial guide. Reducing the size of the guide allows closer proximity of two shade tabs to the patient's tooth, and this often clarifies the selection procedure.

By using daylight and artificial colour match illuminants more predictable results are assured. Utilizing light sources with slight differences in colour temperatures will allow the various colours within the tooth to become more dominant, thereby making the observer more aware of the many different hues that may be present within the tooth.

2.2 Shade Selection and Completion of Restoration by the Technician

Of prime importance to the patient is the aesthetic quality of the restoration, for this reason good co-operation between dentist and technician is essential.

Many technicians have only the opportunity to visualize their work as crowns on plaster casts. If the restoration can be seen by the technician when it is seated in the mouth then a more aesthetic and predictable result will be achieved.

The author has developed a system with his dentist whereby the patient is required to visit the laboratory on two separate occasions.

Initial Visit

An initial visit by the patient to the laboratory is essential for both ceramist and patient to discuss the possible result of the treatment. Very often a person's expectations cannot be written as a laboratory instruction. The personal contact between the creator of the restored dentition and the patient is important if the full expectations of the patient are to be realized.

At this time colour selection procedures are used to note basic shade, depth of chroma, translucency of the enamel and any other criteria necessary to build the restoration.

2.3 Tooth Guides

The development of a system relying on a variety of custom tooth guides will help to improve an understanding of the many essential criteria of tooth character that help to produce an acceptable result.

Existing commercially available guides provide limited information, particularly in the incisal region where translucency, mamelons and halo effects are important if subtle variations in shade and character are to compliment the basic shade to create individuality.

Custom-made guides are important to provide the necessary records and should include the following (figs 13 to 17):
a) Enamel[4]
b) High Chroma Dentine[5]
c) Texture/Lustre[6, 7]
d) Modified half[8]

The Vita custom guide is useful for the speedy construction of an individual guide or the fabrication of a custom shade guide.

A useful commercial guide is the Creative Colour System[9] produced by Ducera* (figs 18 to 20). This system of natural dentine colours blends ceramic frits to match not only root areas but also mamelons, secondary dentine and incisal blue halo effects.

When colour characteristics within a tooth such as mamelons, abrasion areas or exposed roots cannot be matched with the tooth guides then a visualising liquid is used to mix blends of High Chroma Dentines and, if necessary, surface stains until the correct blend is achieved. Care must be taken to avoid contact with the patient's tissues as Color Clue Liquid is slightly toxic and can cause a burning sensation to tissues (figs 21 and 22).

---

* Ducera, Dental-Werkstoff-Gesellschaft mbH, W. Germany.

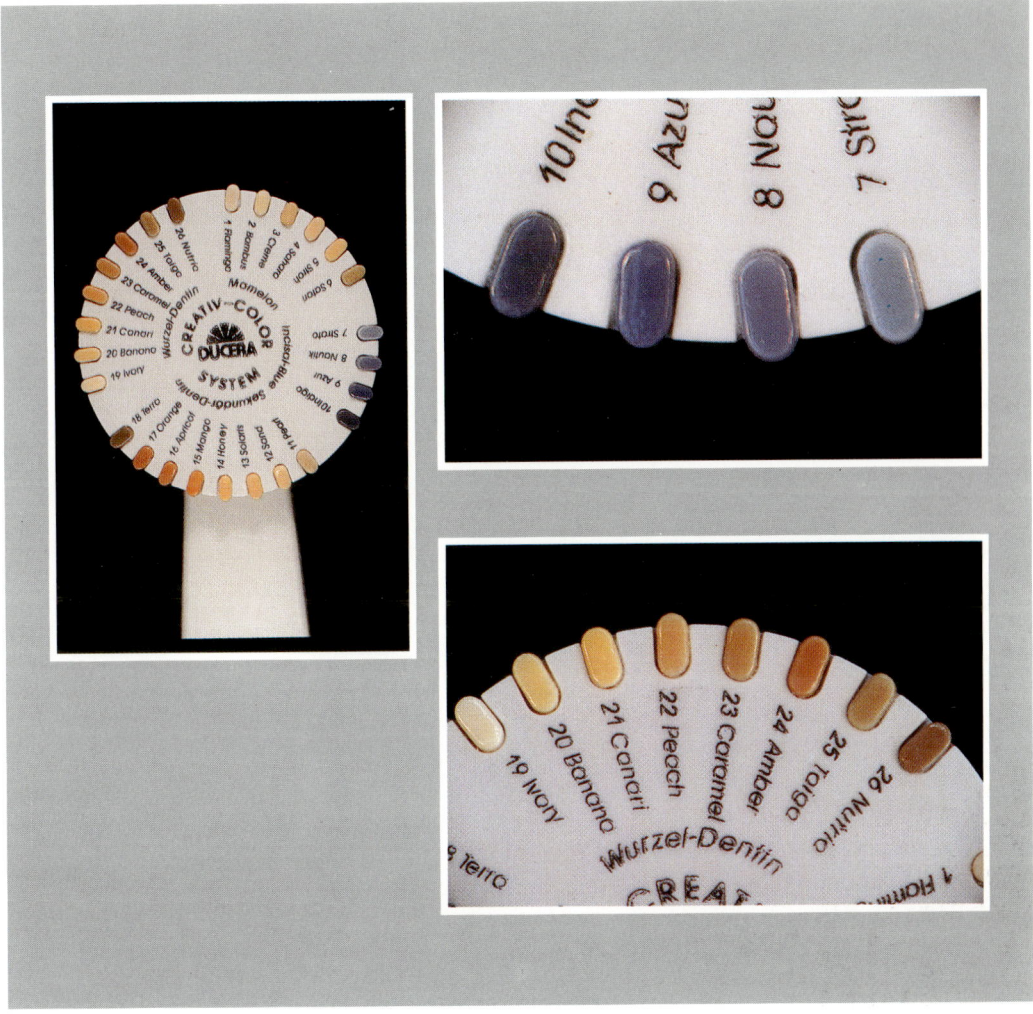

Fig 18 (left)   Ducera Creative Colour System allows accurate selection of many naturally occurring characteristics. The small tabs allow the guide to be placed in close proximity to the colour characteristic.

Fig 19 (right, above)   Incisal blue range.

Fig 20 (right, below)   Root colours.

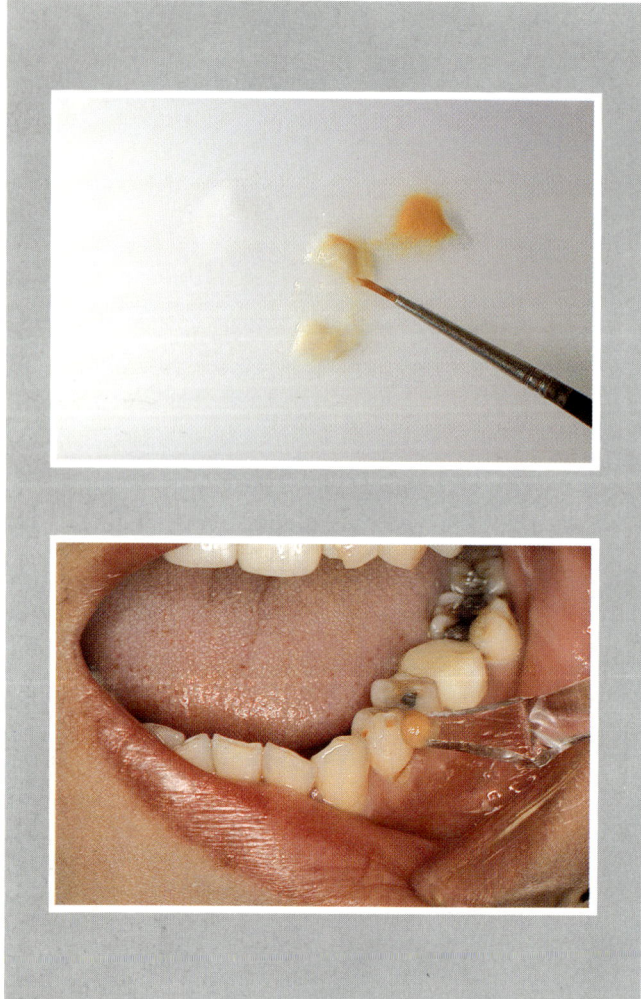

Fig 21 Using a visualizing liquid and modifying chromatised dentines with surface stain to achieve a closer match to the tooth characteristics.

Fig 22 A glass spatular is used to check the modified sample in the mouth. Care is taken to avoid contact with the soft tissues, or a slight burning sensation will result.

Procedures for Shade Taking

With the patient in a seated position, the Waldmann Color-i-Dent II shade selection lamp is used. The patient has the opportunity to view various guides in the Color-i-Dent mirror as the selection takes place (fig 23). Note: The lamp must be held at a distance of 30 cm from the mouth to avoid high intensity light distorting the tooth colour.

Verification of colours under daylight conditions should be made with the patient facing a large window. The patient then returns to the chair for a final analysis of the correct shade.

As both daylight and an artificial colour selecting light have been used subtle colouration not obvious under a single lighting condition will become apparent and with this knowledge a more accurate colour selection will result.

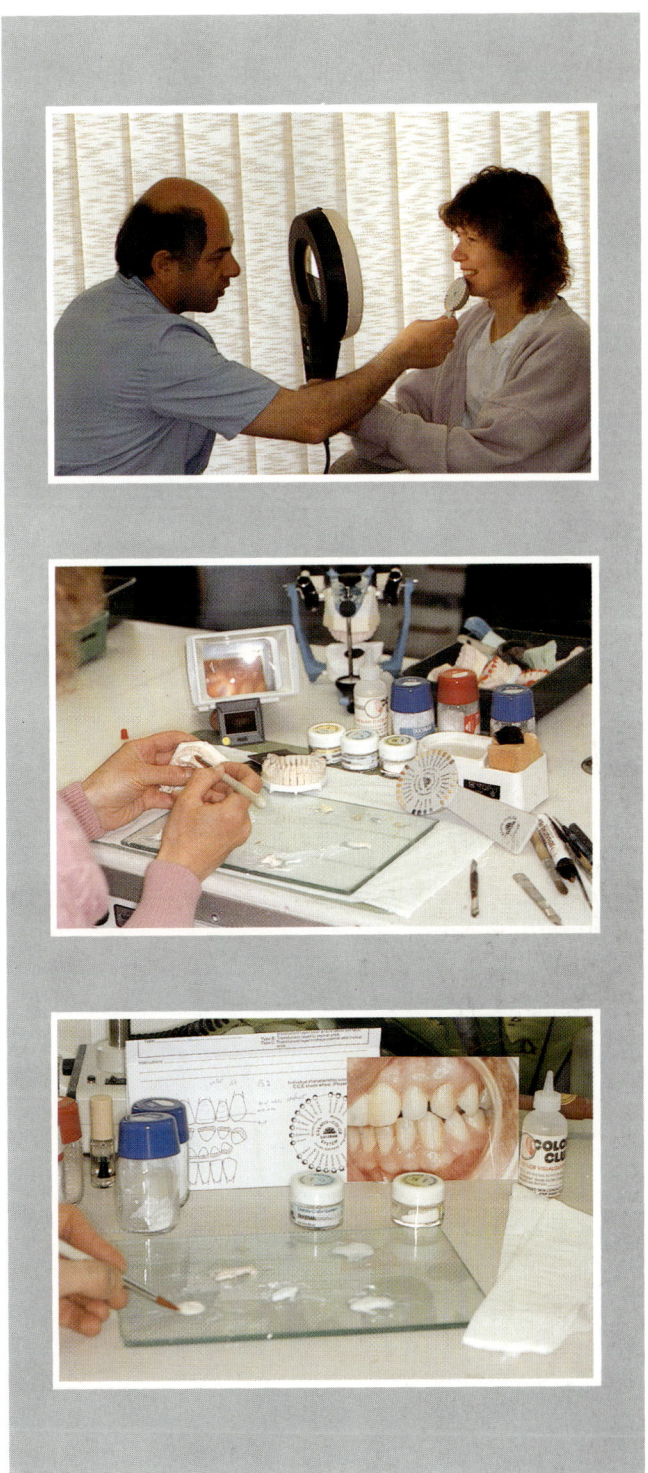

Fig 23 Shade selection with the Waldmann Colour-i-Dent light allows the patient by observation in the central mirror, to take part in the selection procedures. Involving patients in this way educates them to a greater awareness of the colour characteristics within their own teeth.

Fig 24 A viewer is used for transparencies which allow the transmission of light, providing high quality assessment of depth and translucency.

Fig 25 Photographs are useful as a visual reminder and to aid the exact placement of colour characteristics.

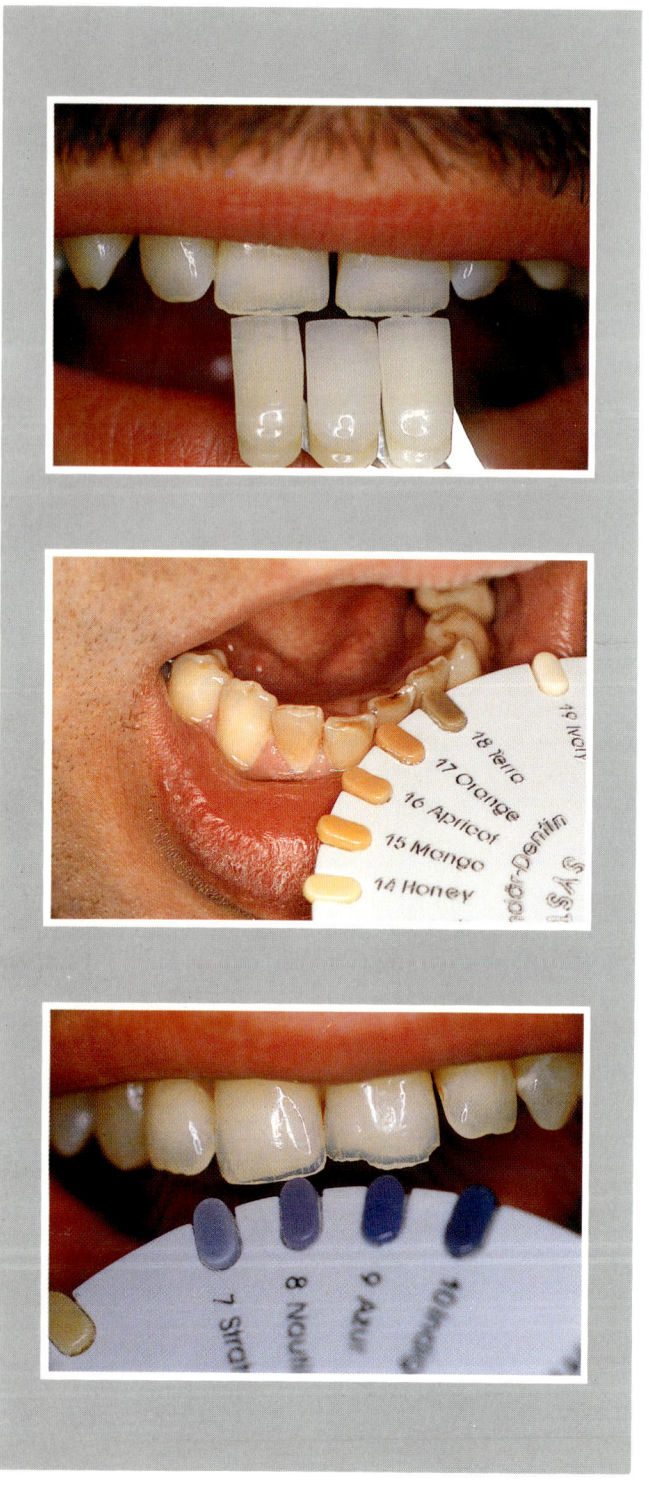

Fig 26 Half guide in use. The centre tab is a good match for the incisal enamel.

Fig 27 Secondary dentine guide shows a good match with the discoloured dentine in the incisal abrasion. This will be a considerable aid in building this type of characterisation.

Fig 28 Degrees of blue translucency vary greatly in natural dentition, and it is difficult to gauge exactly how much to create. This type of photograph would serve as a good guide.

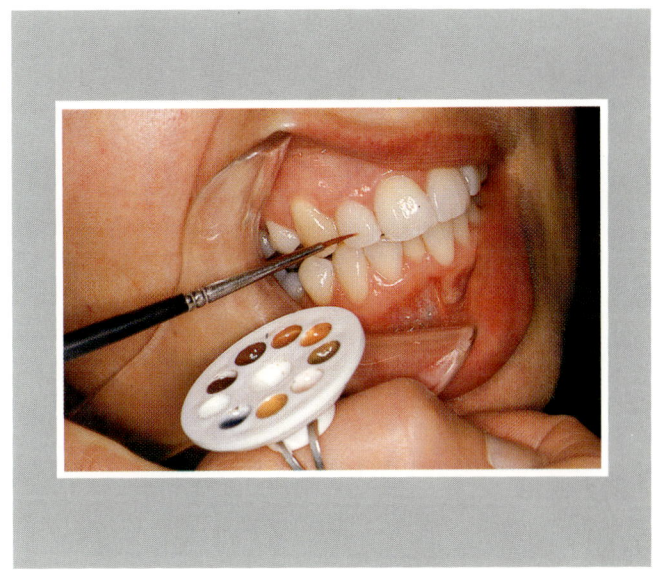

Fig 29 Intraoral staining procedures carried out at the laboratory ensure aesthetic results.*

Working Photographic Records

Photographs are taken from which exact positioning of tooth characteristics can be ascertained to provide valuable information at the building stage. A further refinement is the placement of relevant colour tabs and shade guides within the photograph (figs 24 to 28).

The restoration is made to a bisque trial stage and returned to the dentist for clinical evaluation of marginal integrity and occlusion. The patient then returns to the laboratory where final adjustments to shape and colour are executed.

Final Adjustment Visit

(To be read in conjunction with chapter 9 Finishing Techniques.)

Often the subtle nuances of shade and contour that are not easily observed on the cast are very obvious in the intraoral situa-

* Müterthies, K. Thumb Palette. Dentsply Ltd, Brighton, England.

tion, and therefore final adjustments to contour are carried out in the mouth with the benefit of the patient's personal opinion.

Following final adjustments to contour the natural dentition is dried and surface texture is observed and simulated on the restoration. The crown is glazed in the furnace to medium lustre. Overglazing must be avoided as this will cause the ceramic grain boundaries to fuse together thereby losing their prismatic quality and fine definition at line angles will round over.

The restoration is returned to the mouth and checked for surface lustre, which will be achieved by polishing techniques carried out at this stage.

Minor corrections to shade are made whilst the restoration is seated in the mouth.

The patient will be instructed to hold the lips away from the restoration or, if necessary, lip retractors may be used (fig 29).

Careful removal with tweezers ensures the stains are not smudged.

After glazing in the furnace the restoration is seated in the mouth for final evaluation.

For case studies see figs 30 to 39.

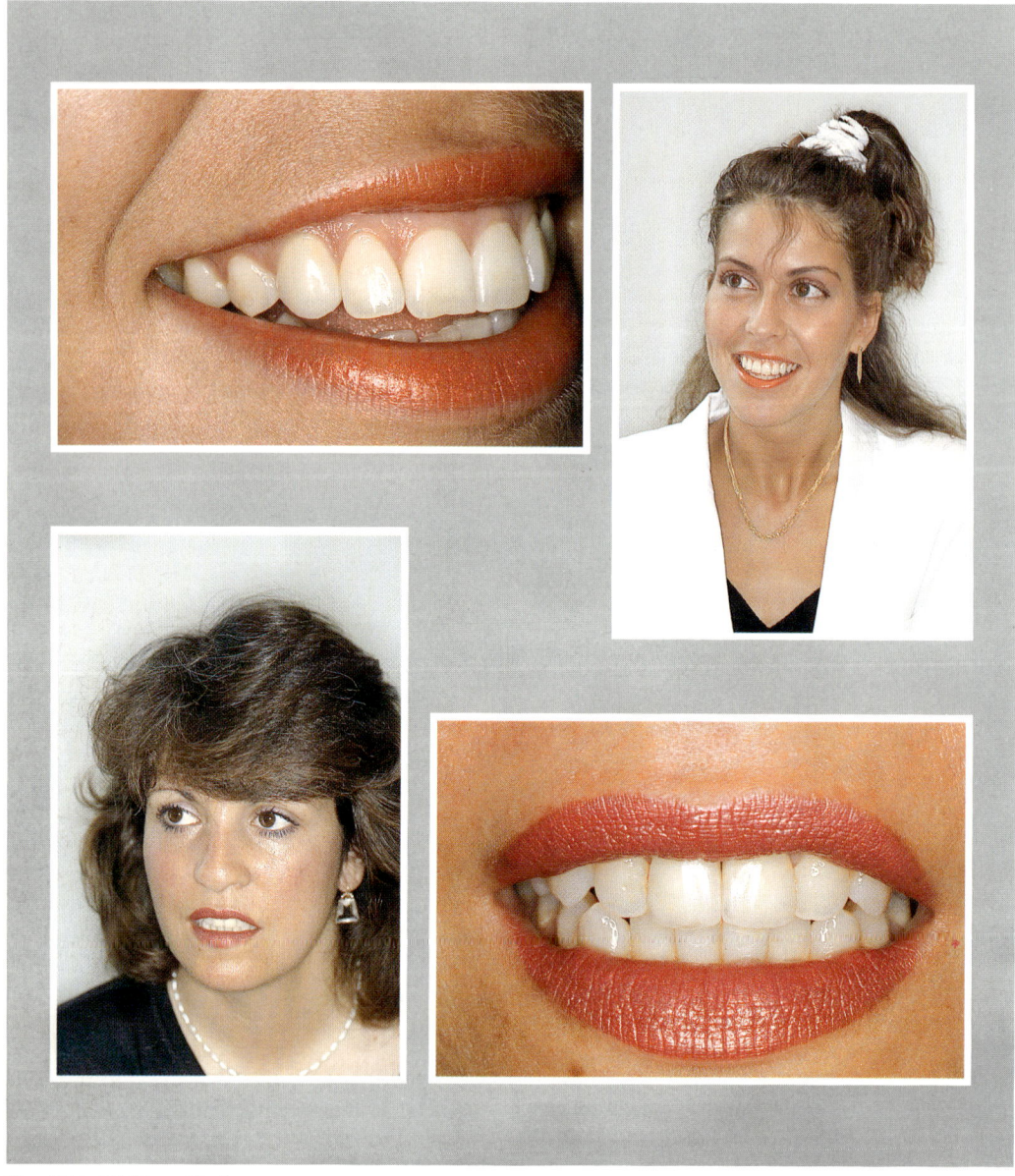

Figs 30 to 39 Case Studies.

Figs 30 and 31 (above)   Metalceramic crown 13 for this beautiful patient (surgeon *Stephen Selwyn*).

Figs 32 and 33 (below)   Attractive patient aged 30 was prepared to visit the laboratory three times to achieve the best result for her two maxillary central porcelain crowns (surgeon *Lewis Simon*).

Figs 34 and 35 (page 31, above)   Mandibular lateral and canine porcelain crowns. Many patients request clean teeth, but it is often necessary to match the staining on adjacent teeth to create the ultimate illusion of natural dentition. Surface stain was added near the gingival margin of both restorations (surgeon *Nigel Head*).

Figs 36 and 37 (middle)   Metal-ceramic crown first mandibular molar, enamel matched successfully to adjacent natural premolar. Metal margin has been used as the preparation was unsuitable for a ceramic margin (surgeon *Stephen Selwyn*).

Figs 38 and 39 (below)   Successful restoration of a single central incisor.

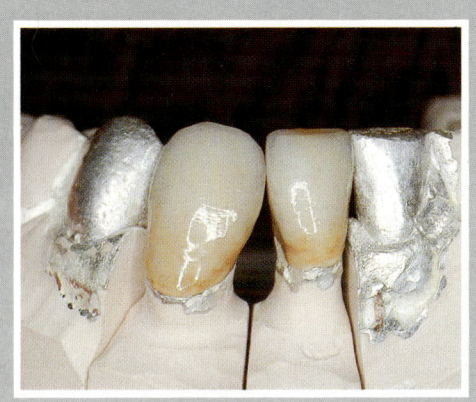
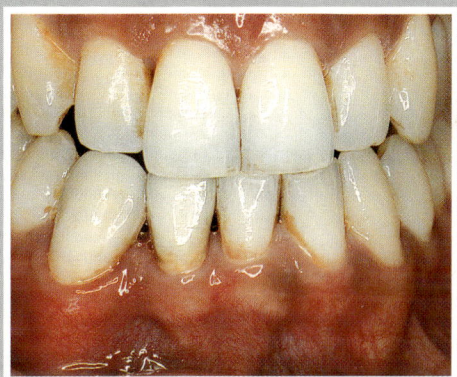
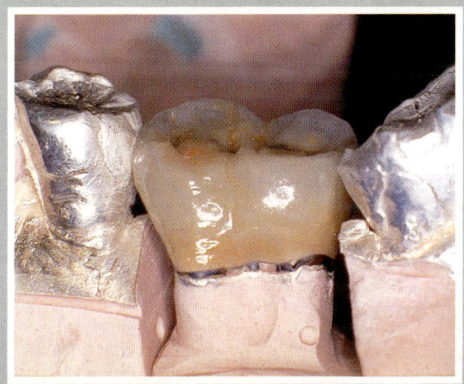
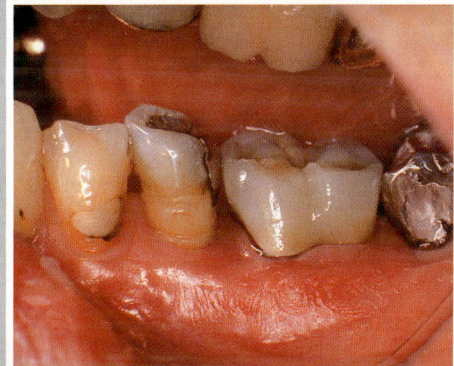
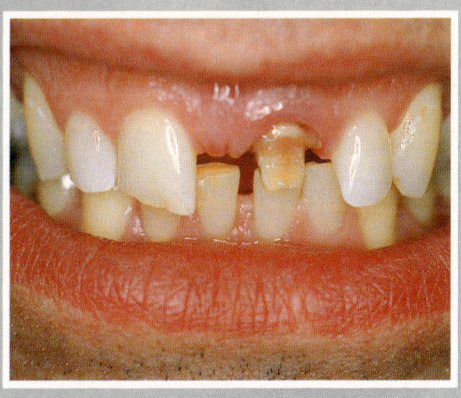
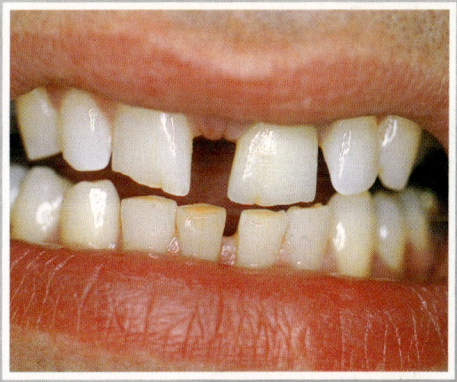

References

1. *Yamamoto M:* Metal Ceramics. p 282–284 Quintessence Publishing Co. 1985.
2. *Clarke J J F:* Dental Ceramics. Proceedings of the First International Symposium on Ceramics. Ed. McLean J. W. p 463 Quintessence Publishing Co. 1983.
3. *McLean J W:* Science and Art of Dental Ceramics. Vol. 1. p 118–119 Quintessence Publishing C. 1979.
4. *Muia P:* Four Dimensional Tooth Colour System. p 52 Quintessence Publishing Co. 1982.
5. *Korson D:* The Simulation of Natural Tooth Colours in the Ceramo-Metal System with Highly Chromatised Dentine Powders. p 453–456 QDT 7/8 1985.
6. *Korson D & Hubbard J:* ISDC Research Programme. February 1985. Unpublished data.
7. *Hubbard J R:* Natural Texture and Lustre in Ceramics. p 263–266 in Perspectives in Dental Ceramics Ed. Preston J. D. Quintessence Publishing Co. 1988.
8. *Vryonis P:* Perspectives in Dental Ceramics p 285 to 289 Quintessence Publishing C. 1988.
9. *Hegenbarth E A:* The Creative Color System. Quintessence Zahntechnik No. 9. p 978–991 Sept 1987.

3 Margin Design

Before the ceramist can begin, the dentist must first prepare the foundation upon which the restoration will sit.

Critical areas for success are the tooth margin and the way in which the crown margin is designed in relation to the preparation.

The following chapter describes the varied margin designs in common practice today and the factors which control the design of metal-ceramic crowns to fit these preparations.

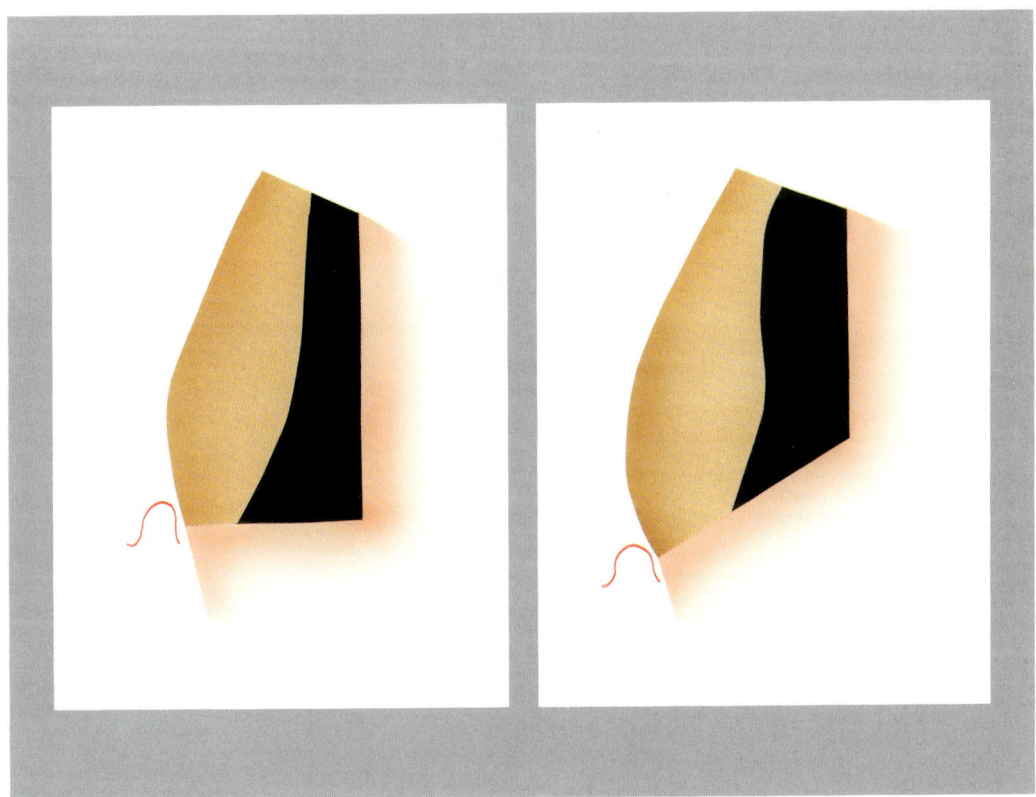

Fig 40 (left)   90° shoulder preparation is the ideal method to create the most aesthetic porcelain butt margin.

Fig 41 (right)   Acceptable shoulder angle, but as the angle of the shoulder becomes more acute (less than 60°) then the likely success of the porcelain margin to resist fracture and to fit with accuracy diminishes.

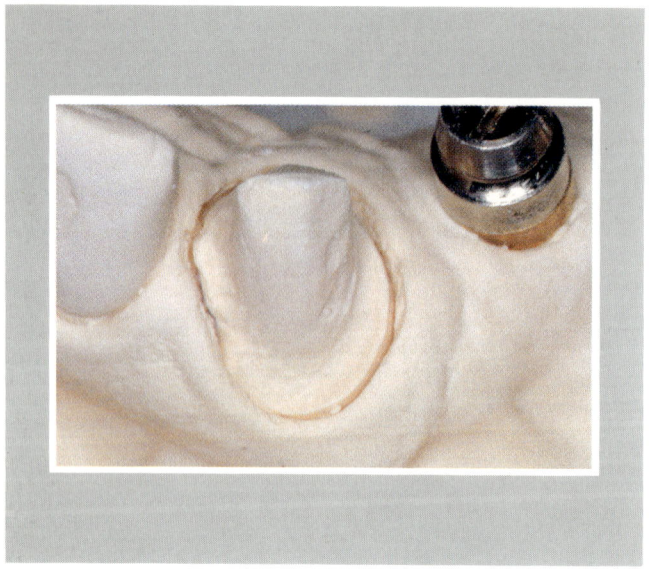

Fig 42 Ideal shoulder preparation for the porcelain butt margin technique (surgeon Lambert Fick).

3.1 The Prepared Tooth at the Critical Facial Margin

Margin design is controlled by the dental surgeon. Knowledge of the effect the various configurations of design at this critical area of the facial aspect will have upon the final restoration, is important for both surgeon and technician if poor results are to be avoided.

Incorrect design leads to poor marginal integrity which in turn leads to secondary caries through the ingress of oral fluids at the crown margin.

Overcontouring at the crown margin in an effort to improve marginal fit often results in and is the cause of many periodontal conditions and unsightly ceramic margins.

Where aesthetics are important the labial ceramic margin which allows some degree of light transmission through the porcelain is the most acceptable method.

Where aesthetics are less important a shallow chamfer, bevel or feather edge preparation is indicated. Shillingberg and others have demonstrated the advantage of long bevels to achieve a closer marginal adaptation[1, 2].

A fine polished metal collar is the most acceptable method to achieve a close marginal fit for these margin designs.

90° Shoulder Preparation of 1 mm width and with a crisp marginal edge is the ideal for the porcelain butt margin technique. Slight lessening of the angle to 60° is acceptable (figs 40 to 42) but the smaller the angle the more fragile the margin will become. Long thin extensions of porcelain are almost certain to fracture and are difficult to construct with accuracy of fit.[3, 4] Invariably technicians faced with awkward margins of this description will need to overcontour the porcelain in this area.

The Deep Chamfer of 1 mm in depth may provide an alternative to the shoulder preparation, although the lack of reinforcement of the metal substrate provided by the shoulder preparation at the internal angle could cause problems in high percentage gold alloys which have a low temperature strength. High content palladium and nickel-chrome alloys both have a higher strength and therefore do not pose a prob-

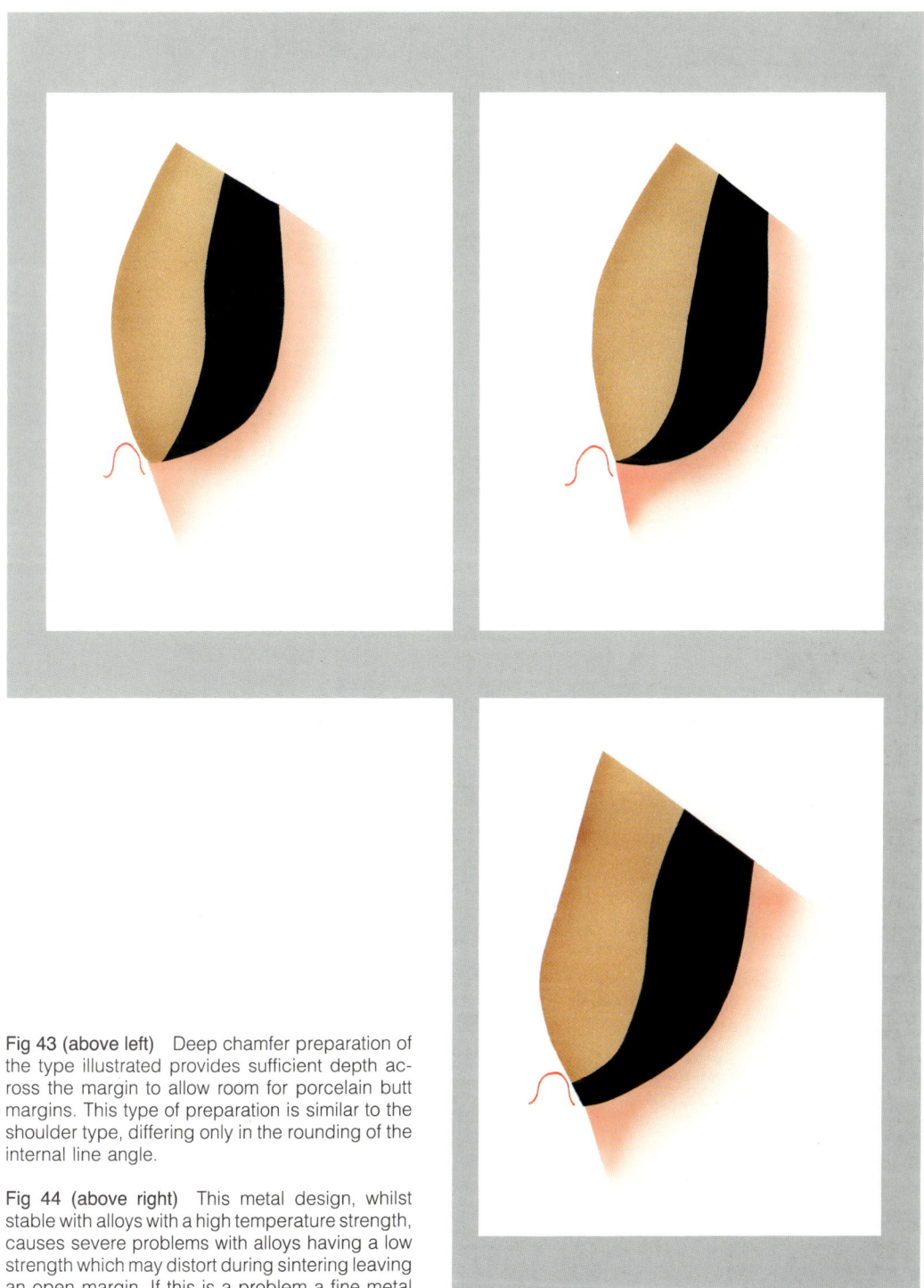

Fig 43 (above left) Deep chamfer preparation of the type illustrated provides sufficient depth across the margin to allow room for porcelain butt margins. This type of preparation is similar to the shoulder type, differing only in the rounding of the internal line angle.

Fig 44 (above right) This metal design, whilst stable with alloys with a high temperature strength, causes severe problems with alloys having a low strength which may distort during sintering leaving an open margin. If this is a problem a fine metal margin is indicated (fig 45, below).

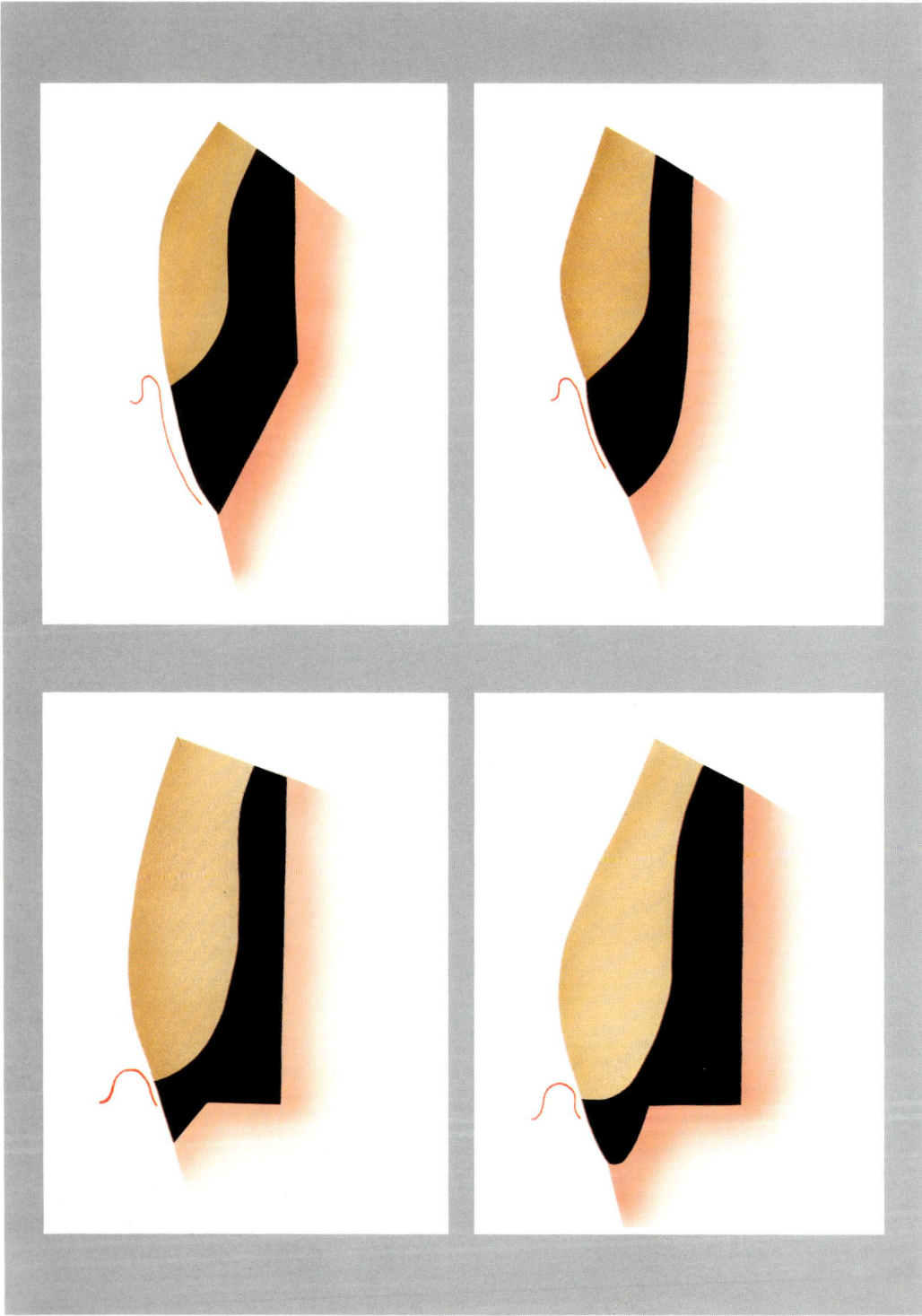

Figs 46 and 47 (page 36, above) Steep bevels and chamfers are not suitable for ceramic margin techniques as fracture of the ceramic margin is inevitable. This situation usually occurs following tooth fracture. Often the margin is placed sub-gingivally, thereby masking metal margins, although problems of the metal discolouring translucent tissue often arise.

Figs 48 and 49 (below) Chamfer shoulder and bevelled shoulder margins need to have metal margins if an accurate marginal fit is to be attained.

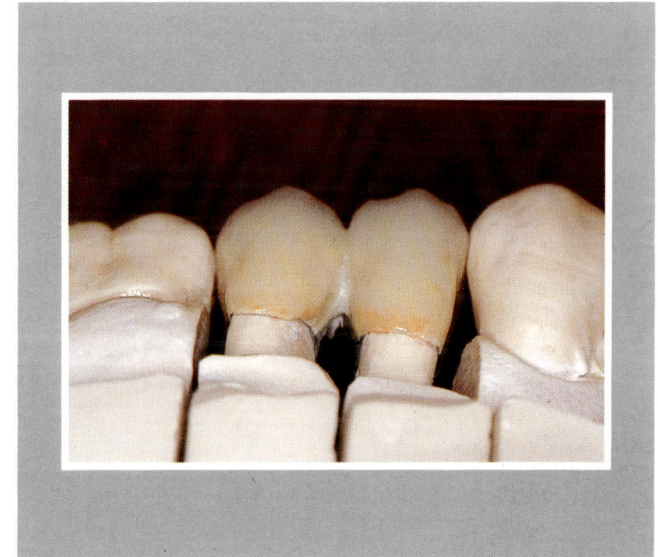

Fig 50 Case with knife edge margin. Porcelain has been built to the crown margin in accordance with the dental surgeon's wishes. The resulting poor marginal fit and thick edge to the crown could create problems for the longterm success of the tooth and gingivae.

lem. The advantages of this design are that surgeons find chamfer margins easier to prepare, and casting metal to fit this style of preparation is also easier for the technician (fig 43).

Shallow Chamfers of less than 0.5 mm are not suitable for the porcelain butt margin technique and are best accommodated by maintaining the metal to full depth with a covering of porcelain to hide the metal. This may prove adequate providing the crown contour allows sufficient room, at least 0.7 mm for porcelain and metal; less space will produce too thin a dentine covering over the opaque which will shine through with disappointing results (figs 44 and 45).

Feather edges and long bevels are contra-indicated for porcelain margins as neither design can withstand the distortions that occur during the sintering process. Inevitably a slight creep occurs during the sintering process, leaving a space between metal and tooth which is impossible to close. Furthermore, a grey line can result at the margin due to the metal substrate influencing the colour of the ceramic (figs 46 and 47).

Bevelled Shoulders and Chamfer Shoulders are also contra-indicated for the porcelain margin technique for similar reasons to those stated above (figs 48 and 49).

3.2 Porcelain Butt Margin

As previously mentioned the porcelain butt margin is the most aesthetic and the method of choice in all anterior restorations. Most manufacturers provide shoulder porcelain specifically designed for this technique and of a finer grain size to aid adaptation to the margin. Small grains packed together provide a more continuous line than larger grains. In addition these special frits have a maturation temperature above the dentine to add stability and prevent rounding of fine margins. A further consideration is the problem of grey shadows cast through the root dentine; where the crown margin is supra-gingival this can cause severe discolouration.

Detailed methods for the porcelain butt margin may be found in the following chapter dealing with building technique.

References

1. *Shillingburg H T, Hobo S, and Whitsett L D:* Fundamentals of Fixed Prosthodontics p 78–79 Quintessence Publishing Co. 1978.
2. *Kuwata M:* Theory and Practice for Metal Ceramic Restorations p 127 Quintessence Publishing Co. 1980.
3. *McLean J W:* Science and Art of Dental Ceramics Col. 1. p 224–225 Quintessence Publishing Co. 1979.
4. *El-Ebrashi M K, Craig R G, and Peyton F A:* Experimental Stress Analysis of Dental Restorations Part III: The Concept of the Geometry of Proximal Margins. Journal of Prosthetic Dentistry. 22.333 1969.

4 Opaque and Porcelain Margin

The opaque layer is an essential part of the metal-ceramic system in which bond strength is important to the long-term integrity of the restoration. Avoidance of bright reflections through the dentine and enamel layers by the use of opaque colour intensifiers is necessary.

Complete porcelain margins are the most aesthetic and therefore this type of margin is employed whenever appearance is important.

4.1 Controlling Reflective Opaques

Modification of the opaque layer to better control opaque reflection through the dentine and enamel layers has been practised for many years. Ceramic manufacturers provide coloured opaque intensifiers for this purpose. Intended for adding in small quantities to the basic shade to influence the colour, they usually include white, yellow, brown, green, blue and grey.

A subtle blending of colour is made possible by painting the intensifier directly onto the pre-sintered opaque in the same way as surface stains are applied using water as the carrier medium (see Opaque Shading).

Natural colour opaque intensifiers

An improvement on these systems would be the introduction of colour intensifiers formulated to match the basic hue range in the shade guides. This is particularly important at the margin and where long labial extentions in areas of gingival recession give rise to thin sections of porcelain. It is important that such places have the core porcelain matched in colour to the overlying dentine as overall thicknesses are reduced in this region. In most situations a shoulder margin width of 1 mm will allow 0.6 mm overlying dentine. However, often where there are chamfer preparations, and in cases when the preparation extends apically, there is insufficient room to create a full 1 mm width for metal and porcelain and then the total crown thickness may be reduced to 0.7 mm or even less. With minimal metal thickness of 0.2 mm and minimal opaque thickness of 0.2 mm it can be seen that only 0.3 mm is available for dentine porcelain.

In addition the possible need to simulate root colours makes it necessary to match the opaque to the darker colour.

Because of these problems the development by ceramic manufacturers of coloured opaques which more closely match both shade guide and root areas would be of great advantage in areas at the crown margin.

Application and Sintering of the Opaque Slurry

Maximum bond strength can only be achieved by full maturation of the core porcelain. However, sintering at this temperature can cause problems with gassing and sintering contraction therefore the core is first applied in a thin slurry and sintered 40°C above the manufacturer's recommended temperature to ensure a good bond between metal and opaque.

4.2 Application of the Covering Opaque Layer

The preferred method is to apply the covering opaque layer to the metal substrate whilst seated upon its die(s) and to carry the opaque to the tooth margin. For this reason the die margin is sealed with two coats of Seal-It stone sealer, preferred because it dries with very little residue.

Application of the opaque is carried out after the die margin has been painted with a porcelain release agent. A No. 8 brush is used to achieve a thin even coat of 0.2 mm, which will effectively mask the metal. Should the same hue but a lower value be required, a thinner covering of opaque may be applied allowing some greyness from the metal to show through.

To further increase the sintering temperature Duceram Jacket Opaque material may be mixed 1 : 1 with metal ceramic opaque.

Opaque shading

In order to create depth of colour and prevent opaque reflections the opaque should be tinted with opaque colour intensifiers. A soft brush is used to apply the intensifier over the surface whilst the opaque is still damp. The most important areas to tint and prevent core reflection are cervical areas, mesial margins of maxillary canines and any rotated teeth which present an exposed mesial face. All proximal walls, occlusal fossae and interproximal areas of contiguous units must be tinted. In cases where there is minimal room at the incisal-facial region violet may be applied.

Sintering of the opaque

High sintering temperatures should be avoided for the covering opaque layer as this can cause problems with bubbling at later stages. The opaque should exhibit a matt surface when sintered. It is important to remember that lower sintering temperatures will not be sufficient to create a good bond to the metal substrate and that, as previously mentioned, a slurry bake must first be fired (see table 3).

Table 3   Relative sintering temperatures for opaque and margin porcelain using Duceram porcelain.

Application	Temp. °C	Hold	Temp. rate °C per min
Slurry opaque	700–990	2 min	160
Cover opaque*	600–950	2 min	120
Margin porcelain	600–965	2 min	120

* Duceram "O" and "JO" 1:1.
Note: Assume manufacturer's recommended opaque sintering temperature to be 950°C, and dentine build-up sintering temperature to be 920°C. It can be seen that both opaque and margin are sintered above the build-up temperature and integrity to both is maintained.

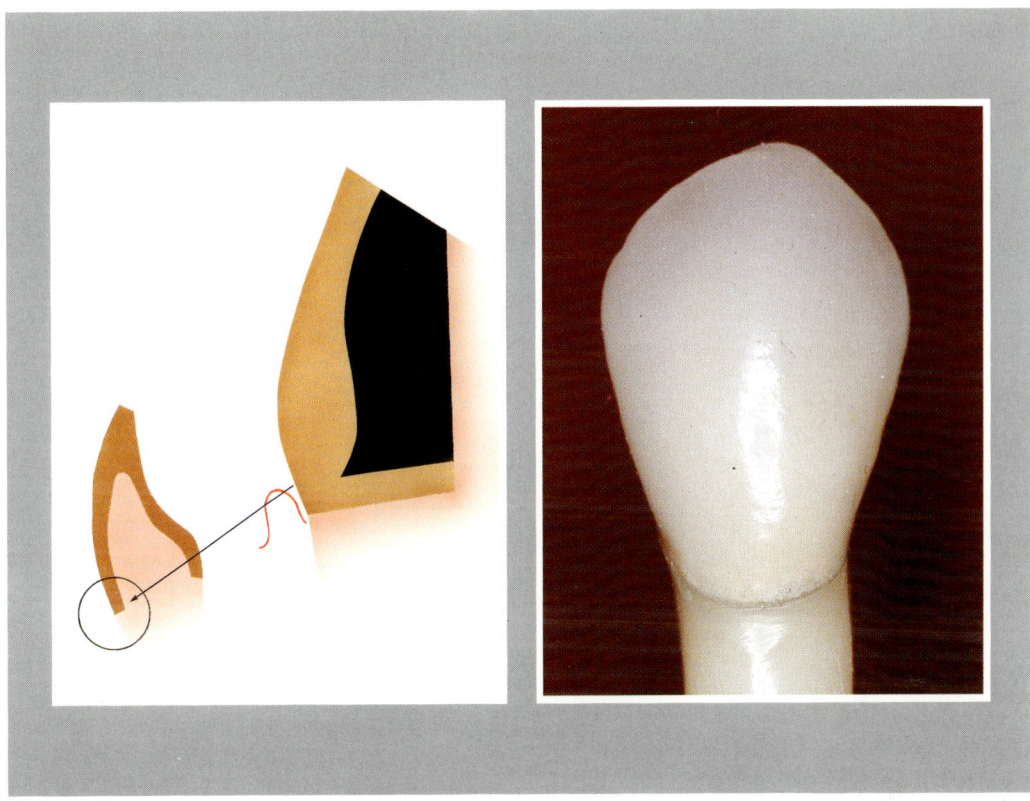

Fig 51 a (left) Vryonis technique for the all porcelain margin. The metal substrate is reduced 0.4 mm from the shoulder. Vita porcelains were specially formulated for the margin technique which allows some light transmission through the porcelain in an attempt to prevent greying of root areas.

Fig 51 b (right) Natural root prepared with insufficient shoulder width. This prevents reduction of the metal substrate to allow room for the porcelain margin, therefore a grey shadow exists and also an overcontoured margin creating a slight ledge.

4.3 Margin Porcelain

The idea of preparing Pyroplastic resistant porcelains for the ceramic margin was proposed by McLean, and the technique was subsequently incorporated in the Vita Shoulder Porcelains.[1, 2]

Various trials were conducted on natural teeth prepared for full crowns with 1 mm depth 90° shoulders. The conclusion of the author is that the Vryonis[3] technique (fig 51 a) has the advantage of light transmission reducing the degree of shadowing at the root junction, this also proving advantageous for supra-gingival margins in the anterior region. In most other situations the technique found to be most practical is to reduce the metal in width across the shoulder but not in depth,[4] achieving the margin initially in opaque porcelain and, after sintering shrinkage, completing the margin with margin porcelain. This usually requires two applications at a temperature 10–15°C above the opaque covering temperature and will advance the maturation of the opaque to a slight sheen (see Table 3, figs 51 b and 52 to 55).

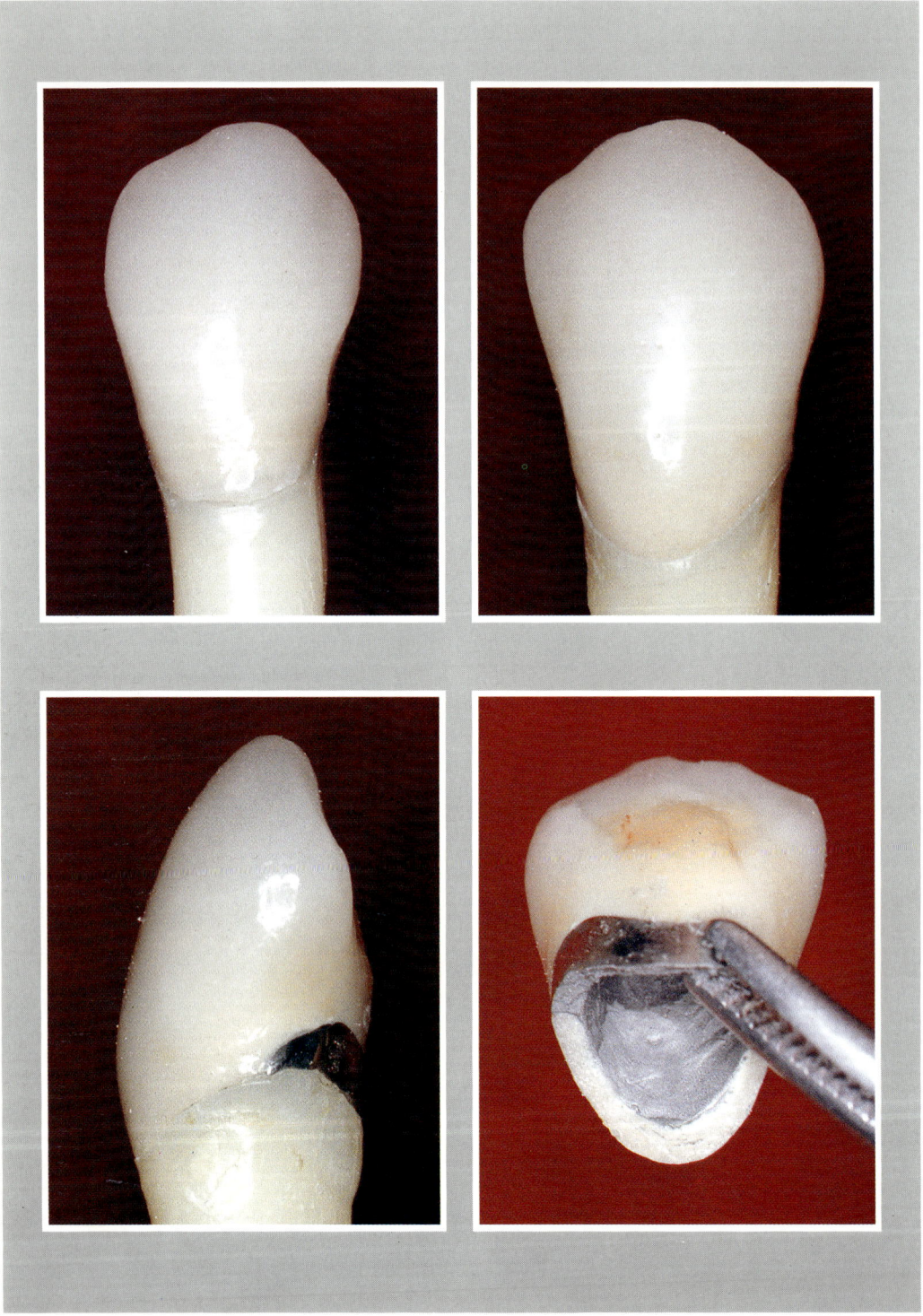

Figs 52 to 55 (page 42)   Metal ceramic crowns fitted to natural roots prepared with shoulder margins of 1.0 mm depth and a 90° shoulder angle.

Fig 52 (above left)   Metal has been reduced 0.3 mm in width across the margin to create space for the porcelain. This is the most practical method as it minimises sintering skrinkage.

Fig 53 (above right)   The Vryonis technique: metal has been reduced both across the shoulder and in depth by 0.4 mm; an additional firing is necessary due to increased shrinkage; improved light transmission and colour match are the result.

Fig 54 (below left)   Side view: labial wall contour in complete harmony with root profile.

Fig 55 (below right)   Porcelain margin, Vryonis technique.

Direct Lift Off Technique

The die margin is sealed with two coats of Seal-It* stone sealer; first coat is allowed to dry before second application.

Duceram Shoulder Porcelain is mixed with Doric Shoulder Liquid**, the die shoulder is painted with a thin coat of Ivoclar[+] ceramic release agent and the opaqued metal substrate is seated upon the die. A thin creamy mix is applied to the space between crown and die, excess moisture is absorbed with a tissue and the shoulder porcelain smoothed with a whipping brush. A slight twisting action will often release the margin intact, but if a small increment should remain upon the die this is removed and the ceramic release is reapplied. The process is repeated until a complete margin is achieved. After sintering shrinkage it may be necessary to repeat the process, but usually at this stage the space to be filled is less than 100μ and so very little shrinkage is evident. The technique for metal preparation and opaque application with a porcelain margin is described in figures 56 to 69.

It is important to ensure the crown is fully seated at all times prior to further application of margin material, as raising of the crown at the margin is a possibility and care should be taken to avoid this. The use of air abrasive equipment with 30μ aluminium oxide to blast away any interfering particles on the fit surface is advocated, provided pressure is kept below 50psi.

Steriomicroscopy is used to check the marginal accuracy at this stage (fig 70).

* Dentifax International Inc., Wappingers Falls, NY 12590, USA
** Davis Schottlander & Davis, Letchworth, Herts, England
[+] Ivoclar (USA) Inc., 820 Los Vallecitos Blvd., Suite C, San Marcos, CA 92069, USA

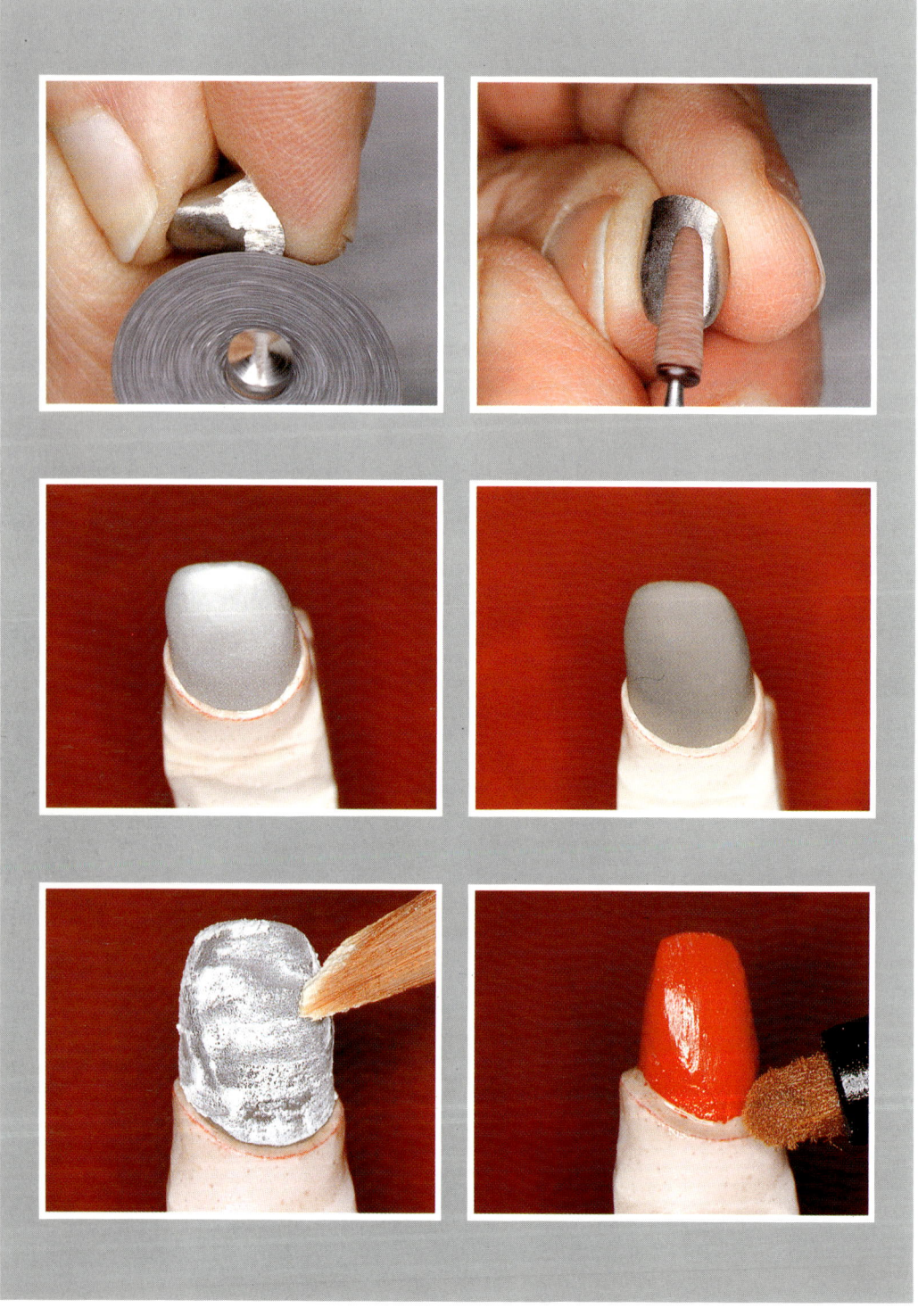

Margin technique most suitable for all cases except those with supra-gingival margin in the anterior region where aesthetics are important.

Figs 56 and 57 (page 44, above)   The metal margin is reduced with a carborundum cut off disc and smoothed with a brown ceramic bounded point.

Fig 58 (middle left)   After blasting with 30µ Aluminium Oxide powder at 60psi, the space available for porcelain at the margin is 0.3 mm.

Fig 59 (middle right)   Oxidization in the furnace at 1000°C for 5 mins. Metal used for the case is Heraeus Alba Bond E (Heraeus Edelmetalle GmbH, D-6450 Hanau, W. Germany).

Fig 60 (below left)   A thin porcelain slurry is applied and sintered at 990°C. This helps to achieve a good bond of the ceramic to the metal.

Fig 61 (below right)   Ivoclar Ceramic separator is applied to the die.

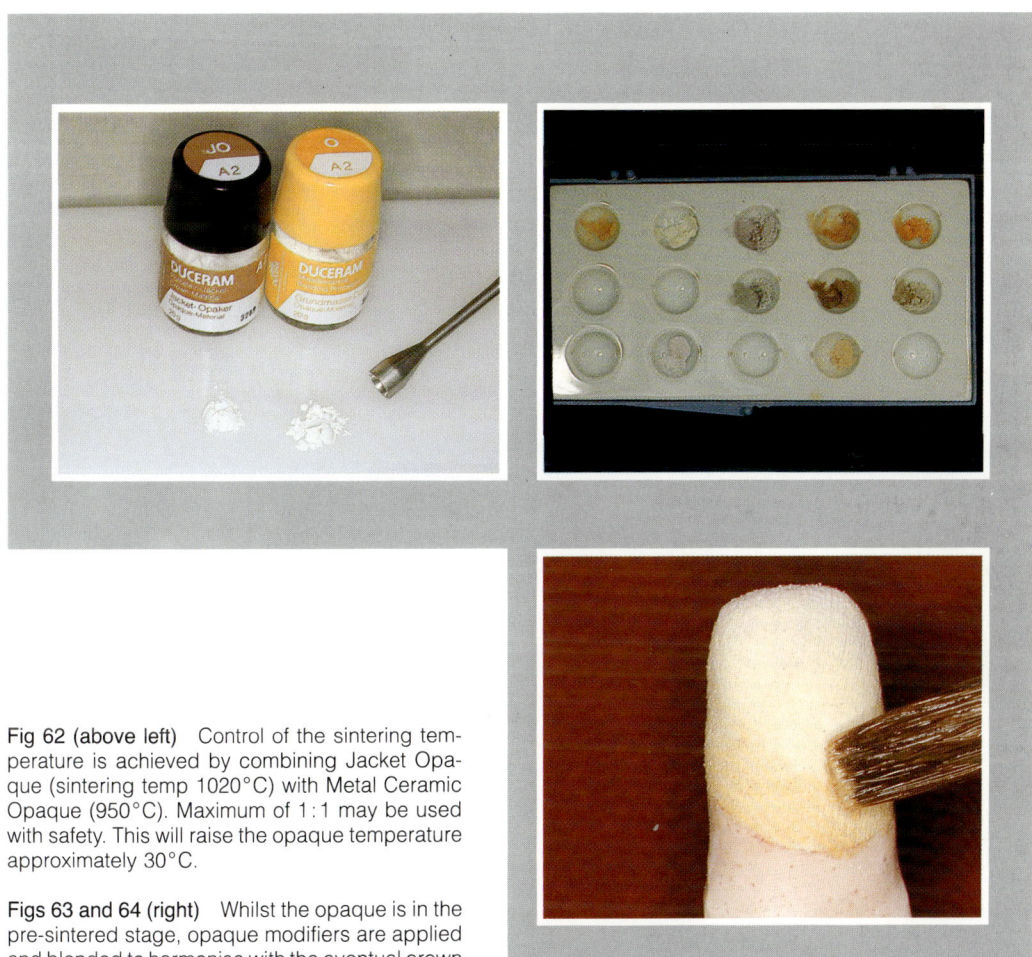

Fig 62 (above left)   Control of the sintering temperature is achieved by combining Jacket Opaque (sintering temp 1020°C) with Metal Ceramic Opaque (950°C). Maximum of 1:1 may be used with safety. This will raise the opaque temperature approximately 30°C.

Figs 63 and 64 (right)   Whilst the opaque is in the pre-sintered stage, opaque modifiers are applied and blended to harmonise with the eventual crown colour. This will prevent opacity shining through thin dentine layers.

45

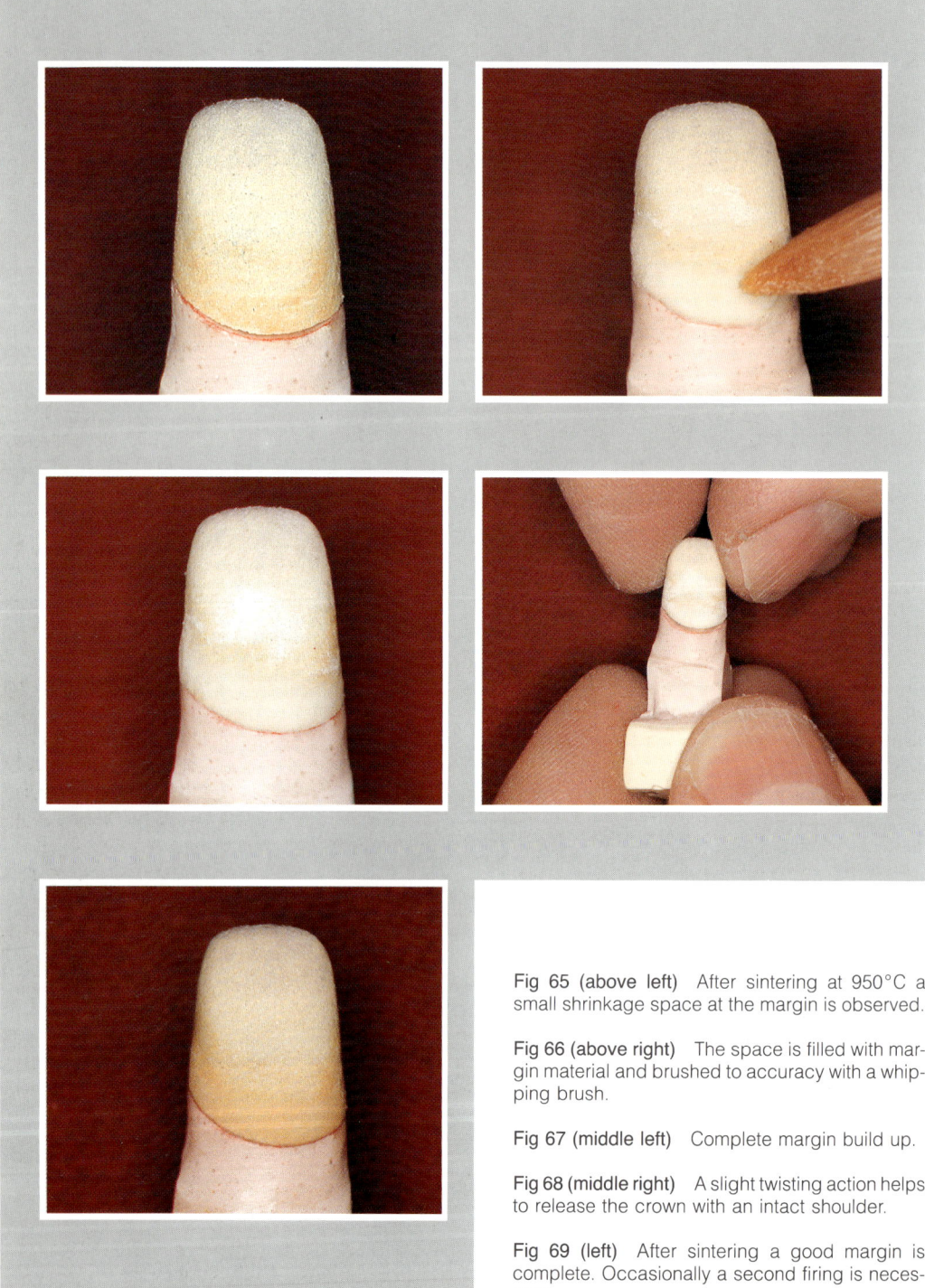

Fig 65 (above left) After sintering at 950°C a small shrinkage space at the margin is observed.

Fig 66 (above right) The space is filled with margin material and brushed to accuracy with a whipping brush.

Fig 67 (middle left) Complete margin build up.

Fig 68 (middle right) A slight twisting action helps to release the crown with an intact shoulder.

Fig 69 (left) After sintering a good margin is complete. Occasionally a second firing is necessary.

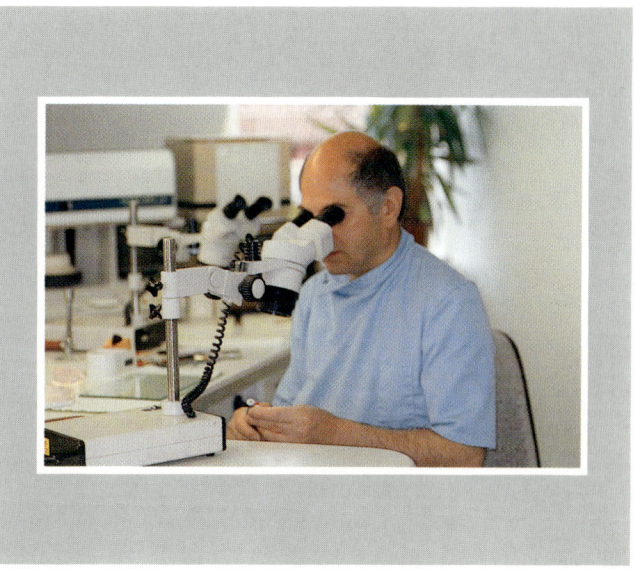

Fig 70 Inspection under a stereo microscope helps to judge accuracy and to see discrepancies. The microscope is used routinely for many laboratory functions such as checking impressions, dies, margin trimming, waxing, fitting crowns onto dies, finish of metal margins, porcelain margins, occlusal contacts and occlusal anatomy and the application of ceramic stains for fine detail.

4.4 Porcelain Jacket Crown Margin

The all porcelain jacket crown is a possible alternative to the metal-ceramic restoration, providing improved light transmission especially if shoulder porcelains are utilized at the marginal area. This is possible because Ducera Jacket Porcelain is compatible with Duceram Metal-Ceramic, therefore Margin Porcelain from the Metal-Ceramic technique is utilized. This provides high stability and is fine grained, providing ease of application and an improved fit (figs 71 to 77).

Indications for use are anterior teeth with sufficient room for adequate thickness of porcelain material. 1.0 mm is the minimum for safety.

Care should be taken to ensure ideal clinical conditions to prevent fracture of these restorations.

Short clinical preparation length and extreme occlusal trauma are major causes of fracture. A complete circumferential shoulder of 90° with margins of 1.0 mm width labially and lingually and a minimum of 0.7 mm interproximally are essential for good results.

Figs 71 to 74 see page 48:

Fig 71 (above left)   Jacket opaque porcelain is built to a small tooth shape to prevent uneven opacity between crowns and to give opacity in the incisal region, as otherwise too much light transmission is possible through the incisal third of the tooth creating a grey incisal.

Fig 72 (above right)   A space of 1.5–2.0 mm is left at the margin for shoulder porcelain and the opaque is sintered at 1020°C. For additional strength opaque may be carried to the margin on the palatal aspect.

Fig 73 (below left)   Margin porcelain is applied.

Fig 74 (below right)   Margin after sintering at 1000°C. Opaque modifier has been applied to tint the shoulder porcelain a little darker to harmonise with the root colour.

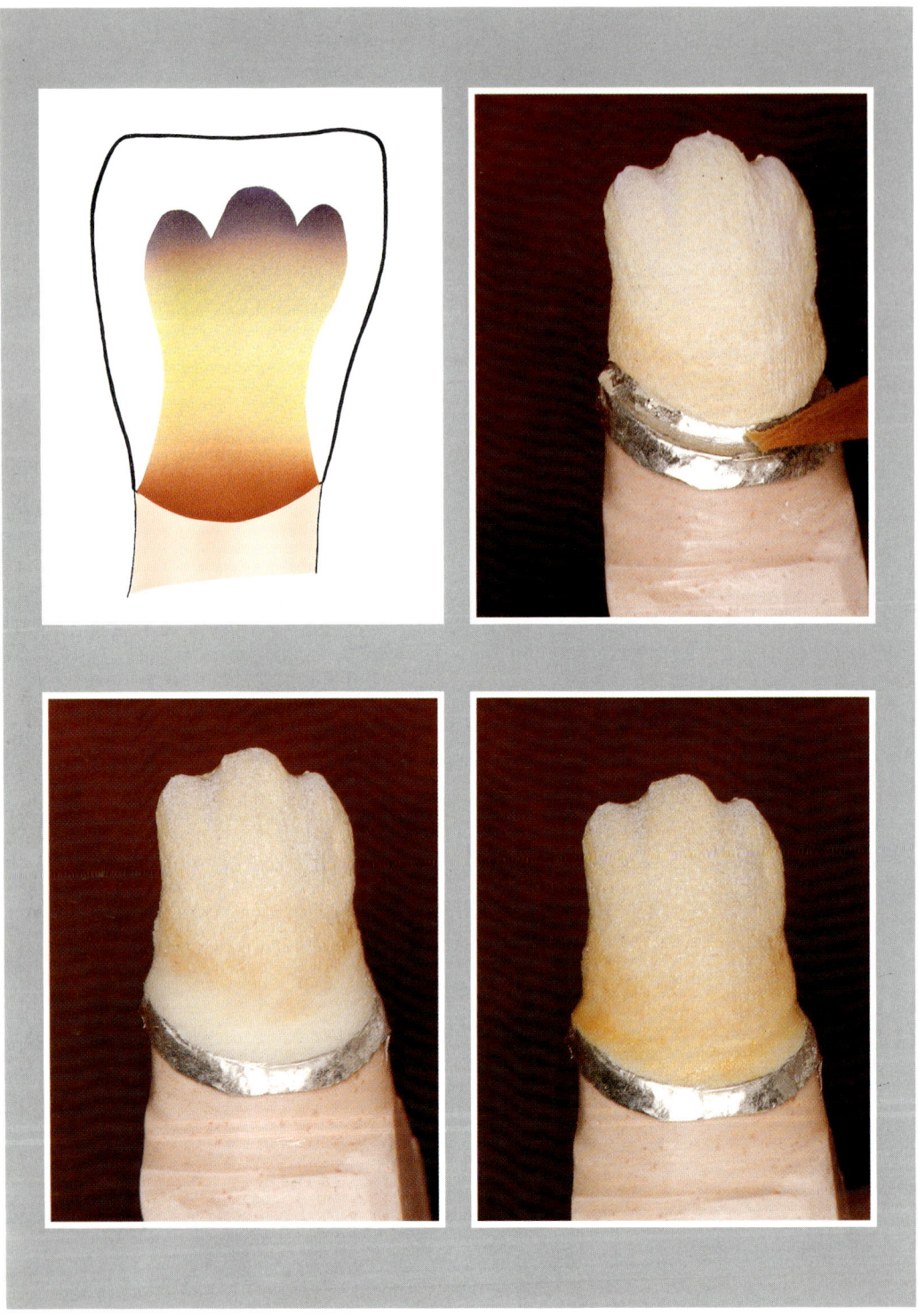

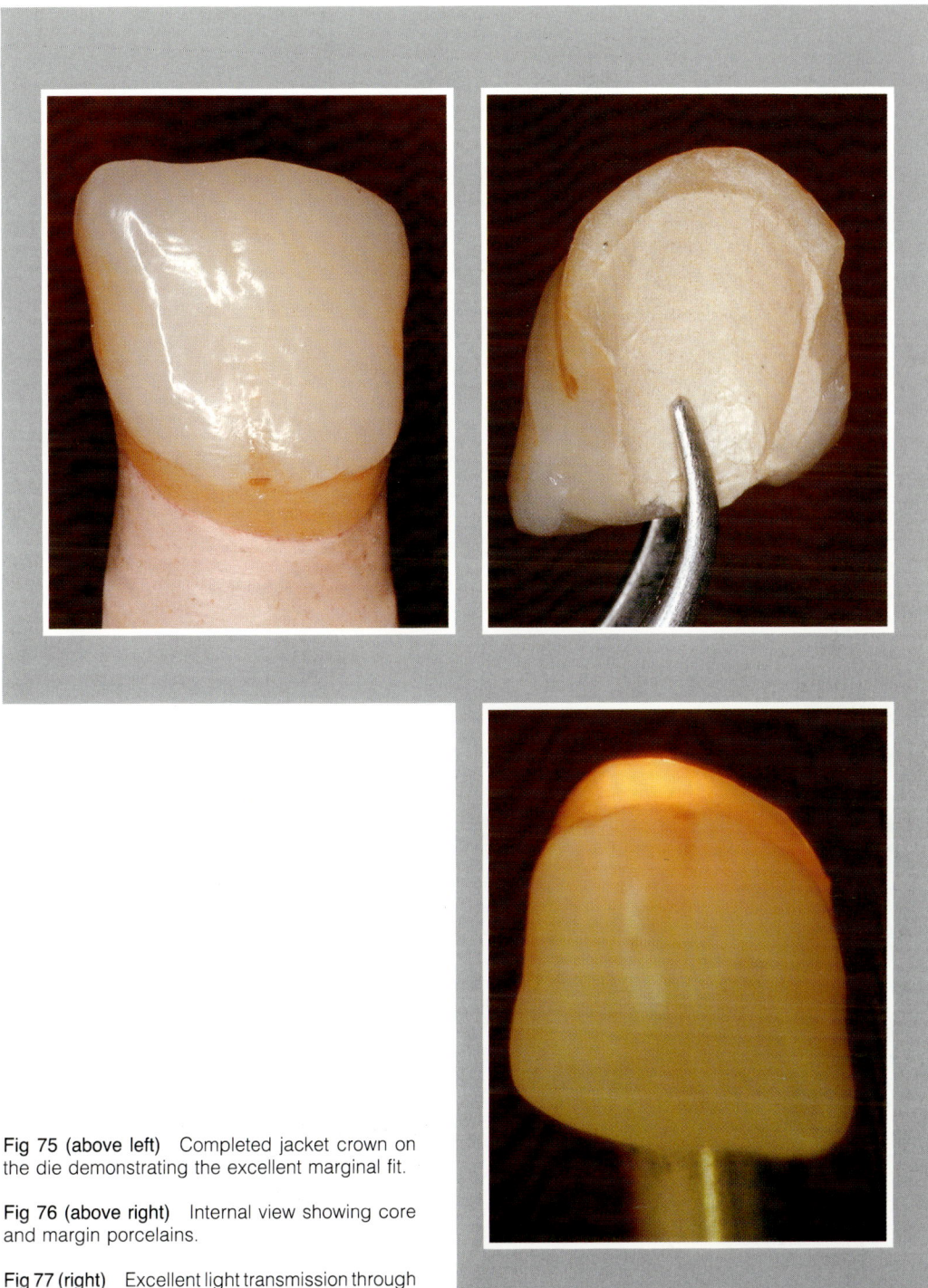

Fig 75 (above left) Completed jacket crown on the die demonstrating the excellent marginal fit.

Fig 76 (above right) Internal view showing core and margin porcelains.

Fig 77 (right) Excellent light transmission through the margin will help aesthetic appearance of the tissues and cervical third of the crown.

References

1. *McLean J W:* Science and Art of Dental Ceramics. Vol. II. p 322–323 Quintessence Publishing Co. 1980.
2. *Hubbard J R:* The Direct Porcelain Butt Fit. Seminar on Fused Porcelain-to-Gold Restorations. L. D. Pankey Institute 1977.
3. *Vryonis P:* A Manual for the Fabrication of the Complete Porcelain Margin. Melbourne, 3000 Victoria. Australia. Published by the auther.
4. *Toogood G D, and Archibald J F:* Technique for Establishing Porcelain Margins. Journal of Prosthetic Dentistry. 40:464 1978.

5 Building Technique (Theoretical)

Dentine and enamel are the basis for natural tooth colour.

The following section deals with the way that, in nature, dentine colour is transmitted through the overlying enamel and the way enamel thickness influences the perceived colour. This chapter will help ceramists understand the reasons for the techniques of layering porcelain advocated in the coming chapters.

The Colour Structure of Natural Dentition

The dentine and enamel frits used to build crowns have an important role to play in the simulation of natural dentition. It is important to understand the effect on overall tooth colour of the degree of colour intensity and translucency inherent in dentine and enamel, and the necessity for porcelain frits to be able to reproduce these same qualities.

5.1 High Chroma Dentine Powders (HCD)

The development of dentine powders which are more closely related to natural tooth dentine is an important step forward in the ability of ceramic materials to match more closely the essential character of natural dentition, rather than an artificial tooth or shade guide.[1] It is an integral part of the building technique, advancing the theory first suggested by Masahiro Kuwata[2] of building ceramic layers which simulate the physical anatomy of natural teeth (figs 78 and 79).

Natural dentition obtains its colour from the underlying dentine layer which is high in chroma. Coronally, the dentine layer is encased in an envelope of semi-transparent enamel which diffuses the dentine colour and also lowers the value. The part of a tooth which has the highest chroma is the gingival third. Being the thickest tooth section and also the area in which the overlying enamel is at its thinnest, it allows more dentine colour to show through a greater depth of chroma.

In the root portion of the tooth, the dentine is covered by a layer of cementum which is light yellow in colour and relatively soft. The thickness of the layer varies from 600μ apically to as little as 10μ cervically.[3] It is this area of cementum at the cervical margin which becomes exposed through gingival recession and is subsequently worn away in a relatively short period of time. This erosion process exposes the root dentine of the tooth, which is highly colour saturated. This is the area of the tooth which most ceramists seem to neglect, since available porcelains always need to be heavily mod-

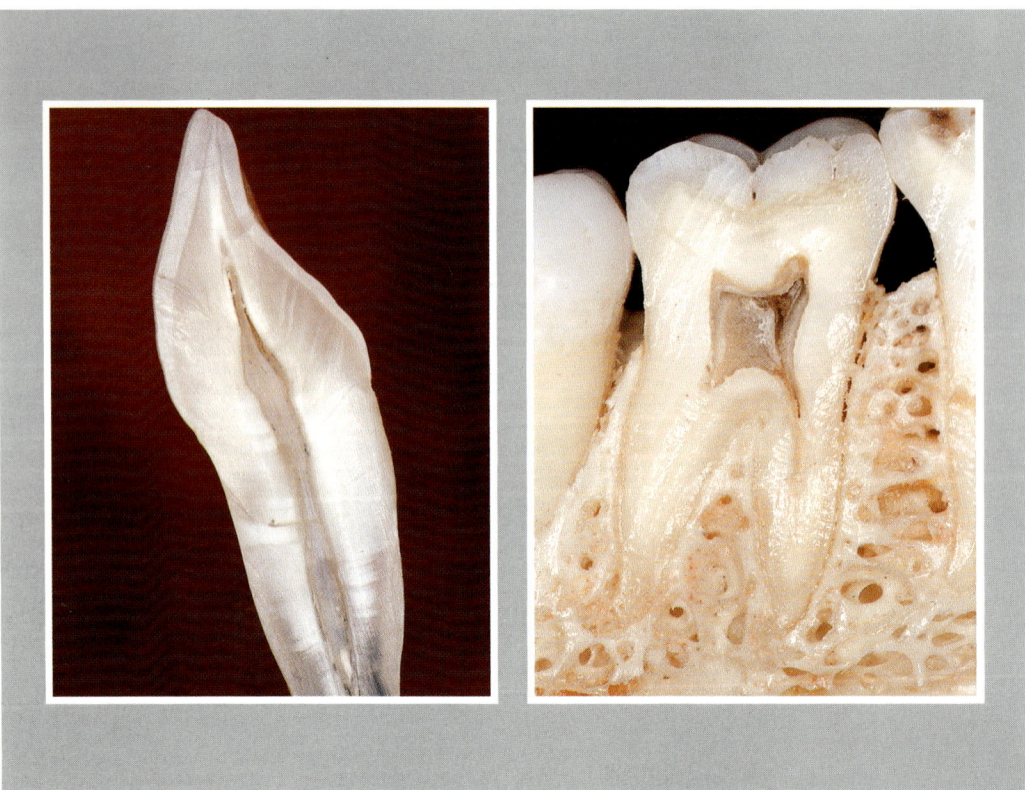

Fig 78 Cross-sectioned maxillary central shows primary and secondary dentine layers and enamel overlay. Dentine colour filters through the enamel and it is that which we perceive as the colour of the tooth. As the enamel gets thinner through age and wear then the dentine will show through more intensely. Similarly if the incisal edge is worn through abrasion then the dentine will become exposed and stained by oral fluids. Gingival recession will cause the root of the tooth to become exposed and the root dentine will be seen, which may also be stained by oral fluids.

Fig 79 Cross-sectioned mandibular, molar here seen in the investing bone structure. The thick enamel at the occlusal table is nature's protection, providing a hard surface to resist abrasion through masticatory action. As light cannot transmit through the occlusal table the enamel appears less translucent than on the facial aspect. For this reason enamel porcelains with a greater degree of opalescence are often utilized. As abrasion wears away the cuspal enamel, dentine colour will filter through or become exposed.

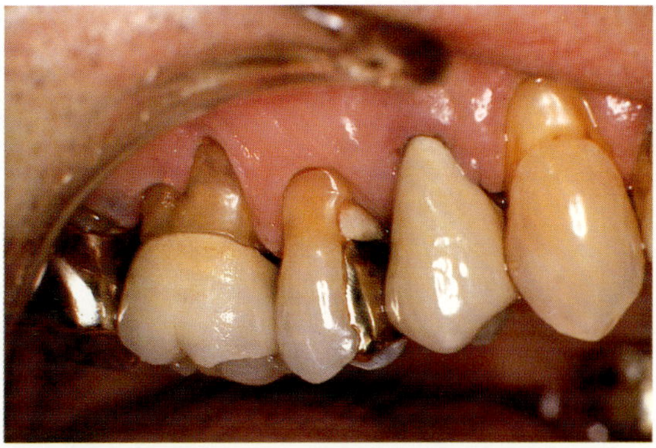

Fig 80 Example of poor crowns. Little attempt has been made to match the colour at the exposed root portion, and opaque is showing through the dentine.

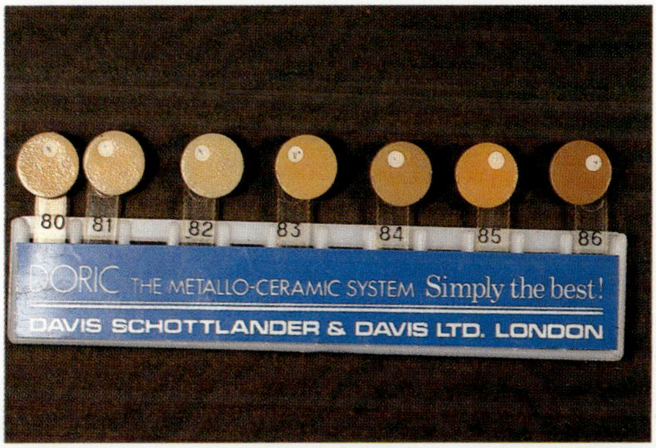

Fig 81 Doric root shade guide also useful as a chromatised dentine guide for building within the crown form.

ified when matching the recession areas in the adjacent teeth. Dentine porcelains do not match the high chroma of natural dentine: because this part of any crown is always thin, a colour problem arises as a result of the underlying opaque layer reflecting through an insufficient thickness of dentine powders.

High Chroma Dentines[4]

Highly colour saturated powders were de-

veloped by the author and named "High Chroma Dentines"[+] to formulate an entirely new range of powders to match natural tooth dentine more closely, and to be used in thinner sections without loss of chroma.

One of the advantages of this system is that these powders do not reflect light, but absorb and scatter light rays, even allowing

---

[*] High Chroma Dentines were formulated by the author in 1984 for Davis Schottlander and Davis, Herfortshire, England, for use in the Doric Metal Ceramic System.

53

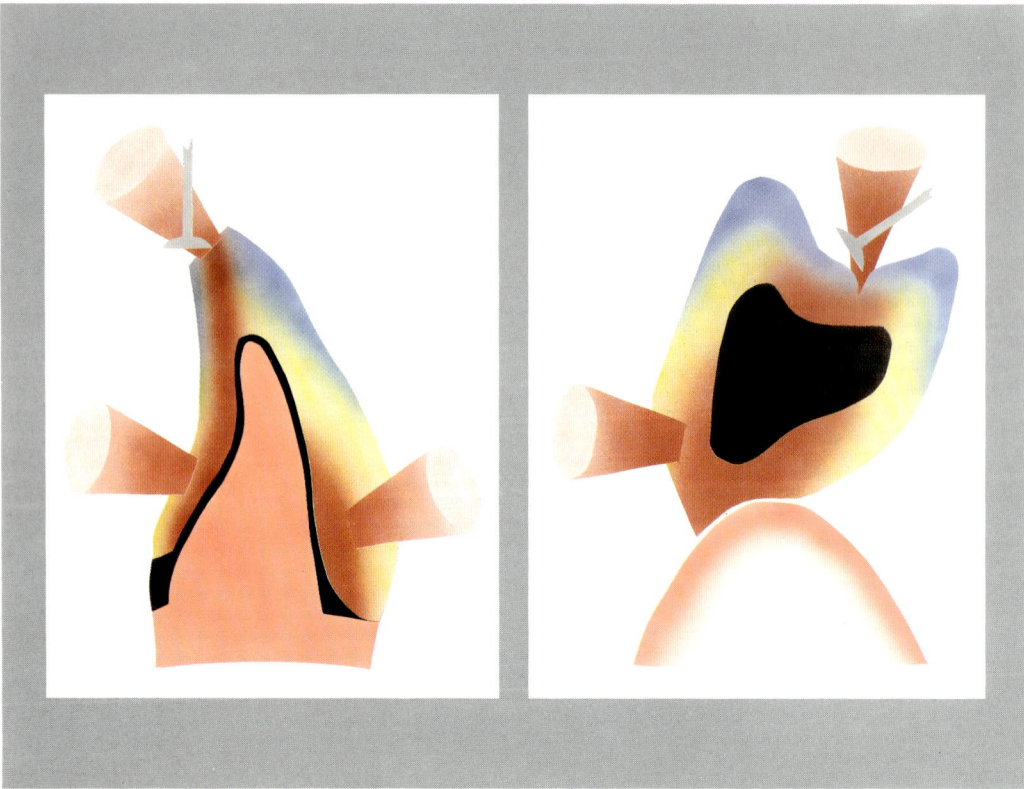

Fig 82 High Chroma Dentines filter through the enamel overlay to produce depth of chroma; when carried to the incisal edge they can create natural dark dentine in areas of attrition. The inbuilt High Chroma Dentine will become exposed as the grinding process forms the incisal edge shape. In this way attrition patterns will form as do those in nature. Similar wear patterns can be created in the lingual anatomy.

Fig 83 In posterior teeth chromatised dentine placed within the occlusal table allows the natural filtering of dentine colour through the fissure patterns as they are formed. In pontic teeth chromatised dentines also help to make a transition to a darker neck formation in situations where the recessed tissues necessitate an extended root shaped pontic, or to match areas of abrasion in cervical areas.

a small degree of transmission which gives more depth of translucency. They also eliminate the problem of a light reflective material being too near the surface of the crown.

Shade Guide

In order to match visible roots in areas of gingival recession, a shade guide is necessary (figs 80 and 81). In development the guide was tested in a survey of approxi-mately 200 patients with some gingival recession and was found to match 85% of these cases accurately. The remaining 15% were a close match and with the addition of a little surface staining became a good match.[5]

A further refinement is to use High Chroma Dentines in other areas, for example in creating more depth of chroma mesially and distally and also lingually and occlusally (figs 82 to 85).

54

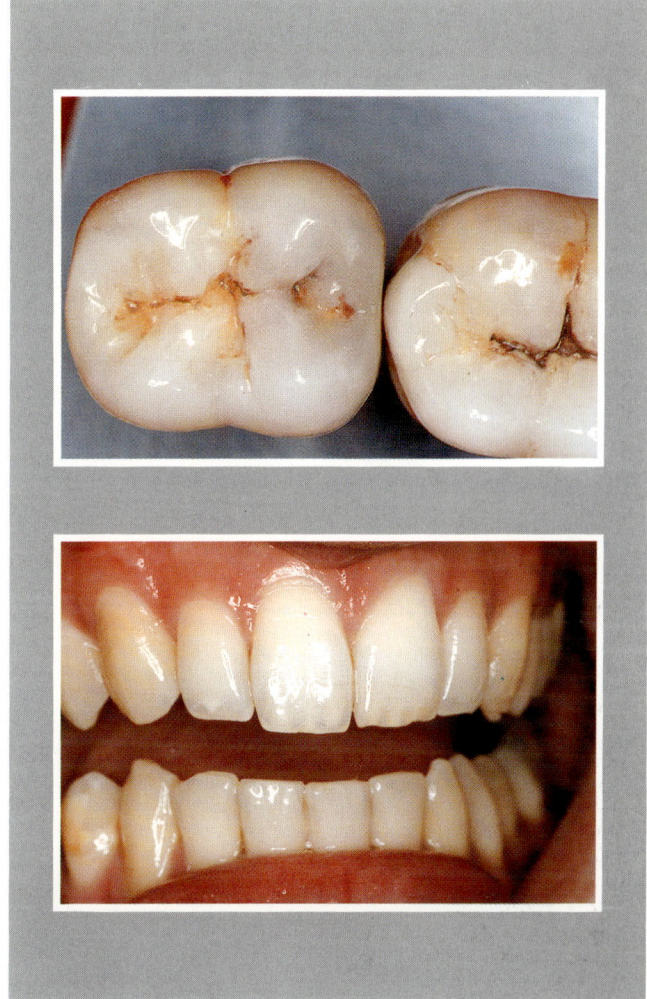

Fig 84 Phantom case depicts occlusal chroma filtering through fissure pattern, therefore requiring very little surface stain.

Fig 85 Example of natural dentition showing interstitial chroma which gives individuality to teeth and prevents a monochromatic appearance in ceramics (see also figs 81 and 82).

Building Technique

The following are some of the procedures used to simulate natural dentine effects.

Exposed Root Surface. In areas of gingival recession where teeth have exposed roots it will be necessary to use the guide to take the shade of the root area. This shade may not necessarily relate to the coronal part of the tooth, but may be much darker.

Opaque layers will need to be modified to harmonise with the root shade which may be totally different in value, chroma and possibly hue from the coronal portion of the tooth. This step will help maintain colour in all its dimensions, especially since the highly chromatised dentine layer in this region will be rather thin.

Building Technique: Complete the dentine build-up, cut away the portion which is to be root coloured and rebuild with High Chroma Dentine powders. Building opales-

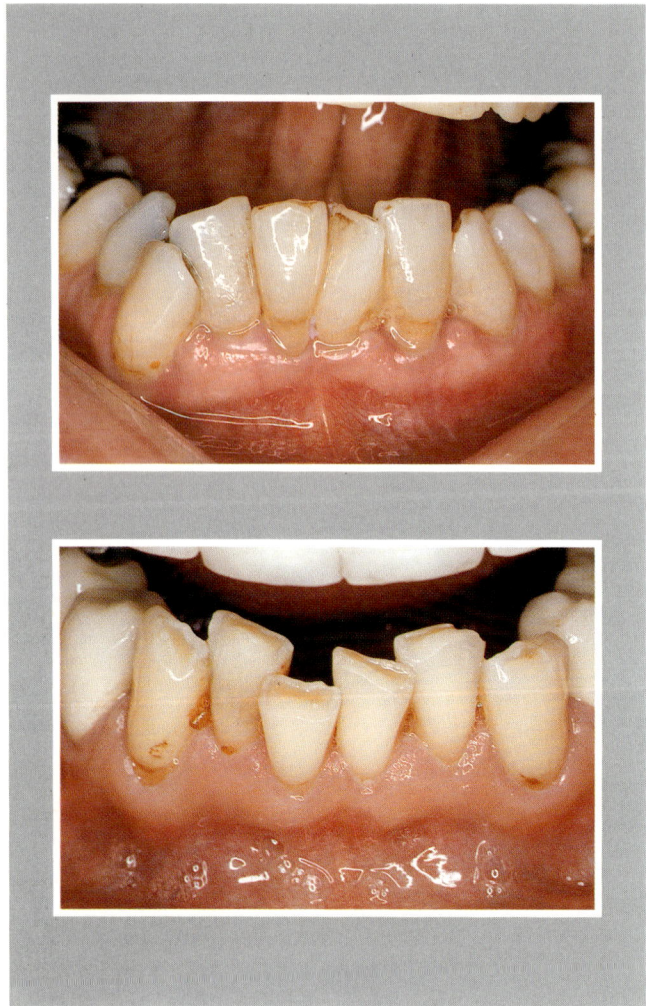

Figs 86 and 87 Natural dentition demonstrates the need for High Chroma Dentines to simulate the areas of gingival recession, interproximal chroma and incisal abrasion.

cent enamel at the cervical third immediately adjacent to the root formation creates a complimentary enamel appearance (figs 86 to 89).

Interproximal chroma. The specially formulated chromatised dentine that corresponds to the dentine shade should be incorporated into the porcelain mesially and distally at the time additions are being made to compensate for shrinkage. The chromatised dentine should not extend onto the labial surface, which is completed with enamel porcelain, allowing the colour to filter through the enamel naturally.

Palatal surfaces. To simulate the darker areas of the palatal concavity, first build regular dentine and contour it as accurately as possible. Then, with sharp definition, cut away the area between the marginal ridges and replace with chromatised dentine. The marginal ridges should be cut away and rebuilt with Ducera Translucent Opalescent

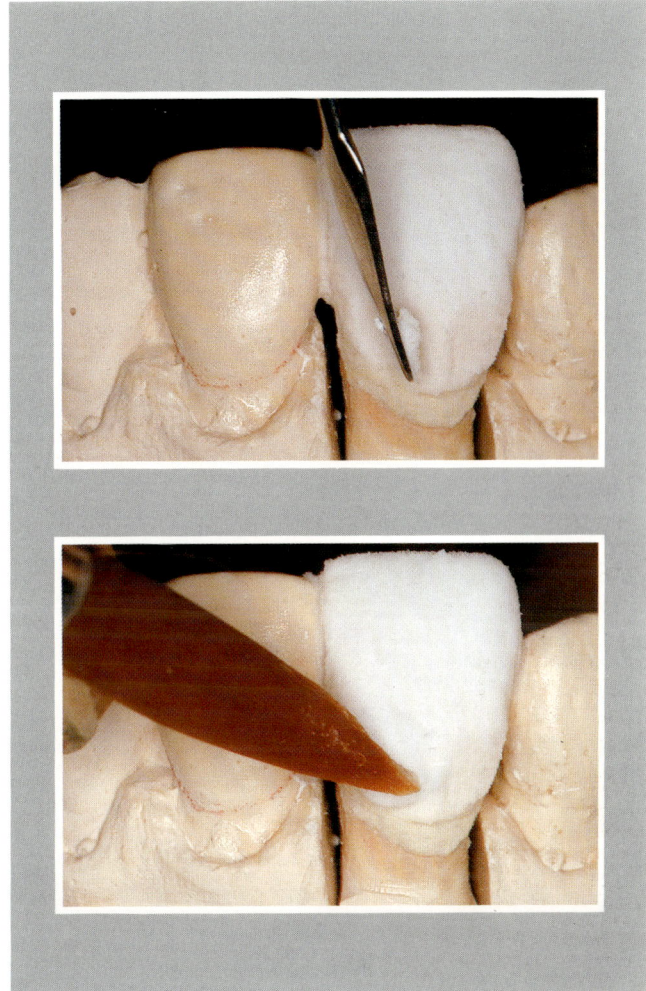

Fig 88 Dentine porcelain is removed from the cervical area adjacent to the root formation.

Fig 89 Duceram translucent opalescent porcelain is used in the cervical region to simulate opalescent enamel in these areas and as a contrast to the root formation.

to give a complementary contrast effect to the colour-saturated palatal area (figs 90 to 93)[6].

High chroma pontic root. The pontic is basically a whitish yellow colour which stands out in harsh relief against the dark red background of the oral tissues. The pontic tooth often looks unnatural because it overlays the soft tissue whilst teeth erupt naturally from within their investing tissues. This creates a problem. In situations where the tissue contour is concave the problem can be alleviated by forming a small root utilizing high chroma dentines to create an intermediary transitional colour, so giving the pontic tooth the appearance of erupting from the tissues.

Chromatised dentines are available under the trade name Doric Root Shades which are also recommended for Ivoclar and Williams porcelain brands. Formulae for Vita and Duceram are listed on page 59.

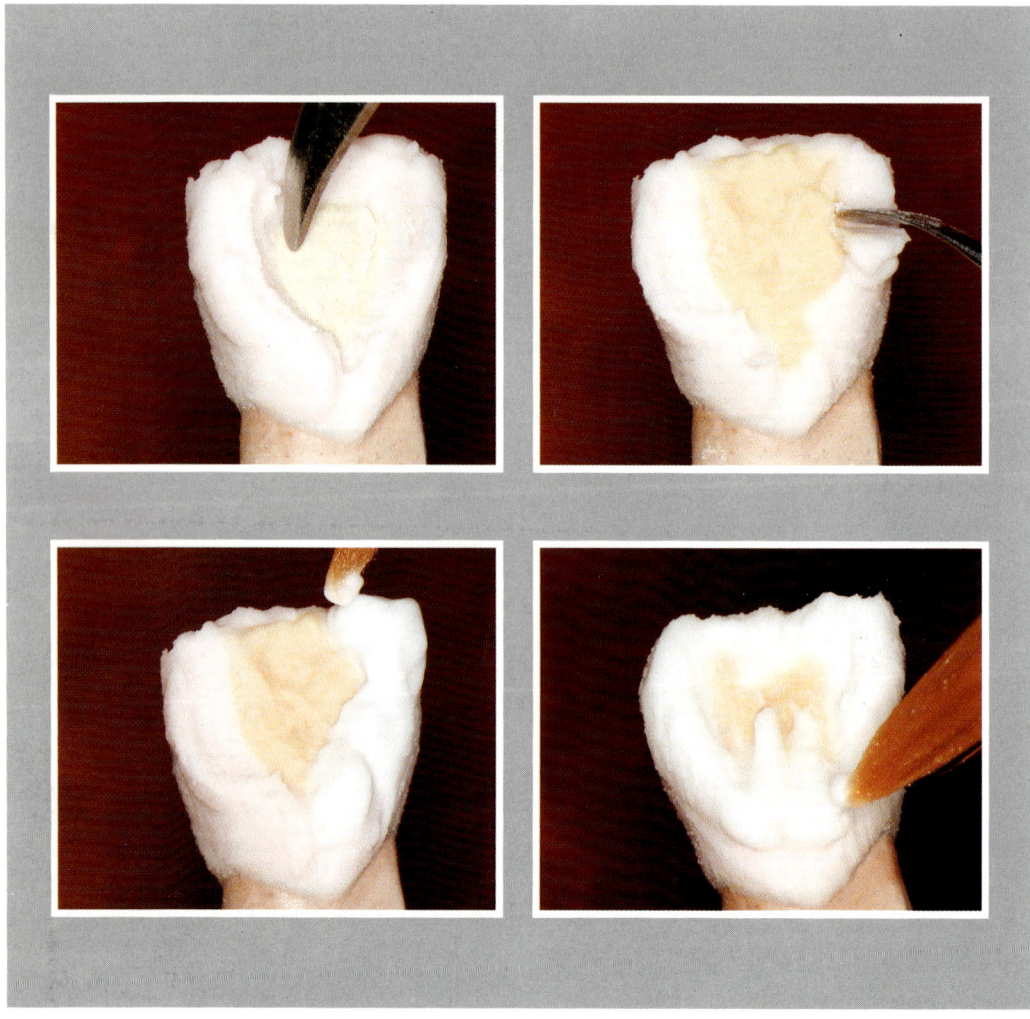

Creating Natural Palatal Surfaces

Figs 90–93   Technique for developing natural colour in the palatal region.

Fig 90 (above left)   Remove the dentine porcelain between the marginal ridges through to the opaque and replace with chromatised dentines. In this case shade to harmonise with Vita A3. HCD mixture DA3 – CCS 22 1 : 1.

Fig 91 (above right)   Remove approximately 1.5 mm from the marginal ridge and replace with translucent opalescent to give a contrast to the High Chroma Dentine mixture.

Fig 92 (below left)   Incisal edge should be completed with translucent opalescent as this will be a thin layer of porcelain and is simulating the lingual enamel plate.

Fig 93 (below right)   Cingulum anatomy is also developed in translucent opalescent.

Table 4 High chroma dentines formulae to match Vita VMK[+].

Shade	To match	Formulae	
80	A1	9 pt	541
	B1	1.5 pt	564
		1 pt	566
		3 pt	568
81	A2	9 pt	543
	A3	3 pt	566
	D3	3 pt	568
82	B2	9 pt	546
	B3	2 pt	566
		0.5 pt	564
83	C1	1 pt	563
	C2	1 pt	84
	D2		
	D4		
84	A3.5	5 pt	543
	A4	5 pt	566
	B4	2 pt	568
		1.5 pt	564
85	C3	5 pt	550
	C4	2 pt	564
		2 pt	566
		2 pt	568
		0.5 pt	567
86*		5 pt	554
		5 pt	566
87*		9 pt	542
		2 pt	568
		1 pt	567

* Most common exposed root area in the older dentition

Table 5 High chroma dentines formulae to match Duceram[++].

Shade	Formulae	
A1	1 pt	21
	3 pt	DA1
A2	1 pt	22
	2 pt	DA2
A3	1 pt	22
	1 pt	DA3
A4	3 pt	22
	1 pt	DA4
B1	1 pt	21
	3 pt	DB1
B2	1 pt	22
	3 pt	DB2
B3	1 pt	22
	1 pt	DB3
B4	3 pt	22
	1 pt	DB4
C1/C2	1 pt	25
C3/C4	1 pt	25
	10% dk brown intensive	
D2	1 pt	23
	3 pt	DD2
D3	1 pt	23
	1 pt	DD3
D4	3 pt	23
	1 pt	DD4

Building techniques using Duceram are described in more detail in the following chapters.

[+] Vita Zahnfabrik, D-7880 Bad Säckingen, W. Germany

[++] Ducera Dental-Werkstoff-Gesellschaft mbH, Rodheimer Str. 7, D-6365 Rosbach v.d.H., W. Germany

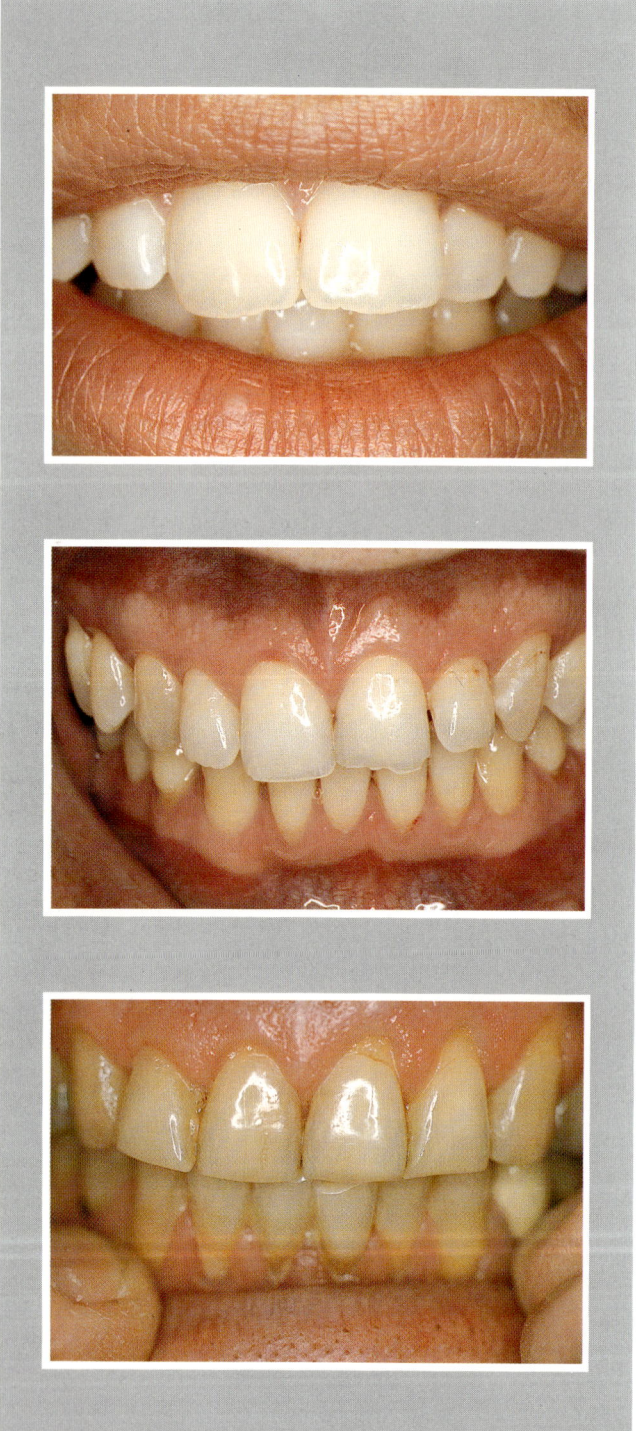

Fig 94 Natural dentition demonstrating the dense appearance common in the young.

Fig 95 Middle-aged dentition. The opalescence can still be seen as a dense structure beneath a translucent overlay.

Fig 96 Aged dentition with worn labial surfaces and translucent enamel overlay.

5.2 The Enamel Screen

Age related differences in the quality of the enamel layer are usually due to the enamel rod cuticles which envelop the enamel rods changing in their formulation[7], and also to the effect of wear and abrasion of the tooth surface giving the appearance of a smooth polished surface. It is this smooth surface which allows light waves to enter the tooth. A higher percentage will pass through the enamel overlay and reach the dentine, allowing the light waves to carry the reflected dentine colour back to the observer's eye.

Care must be taken to avoid applying ceramic enamel layers which are too thick as this will prevent a greater percentage of light from entering beyond the enamel screen.

Young dentition usually exhibits a dense opalescent enamel (fig 94).

In middle-age the enamel opalescence is still present but the surface has become more translucent (fig 95).

With advancing years the enamel becomes progressively less opalescent, becoming thin due to wear and abrasion, with the resultant increase in transparency allowing the dentine colours to show through strongly (fig 96).

It can be seen that the differences that exist between the young, middle-aged and the aged will affect the appearance of the enamel. It is therefore essential to build ceramic overlays which after glazing and polishing procedures (see Finishing Techniques) will produce enamels that will simulate the age-related condition of opacity or translucency.

In instances where intense blue or grey areas are present within the enamel it is useful to use either a custom enamel guide or the Duceram Creative Colour System (CCS).

The enamel overlay varies in its thickness not only in different areas of the tooth but from anterior to posterior teeth. Anteriors have a thin overlay facially and palatally and a thicker section through the mesial and distal proximal walls (fig 97). Posterior enamel is relatively thick on the occlusal surfaces to resist occlusal abrasion (fig 98). This will wear with age and often becomes completely abraded away, exposing dentine. It is this relationship between enamel thickness and the dentine colour showing through that is important in the building of ceramic teeth. High Chroma Dentines are useful when strong colours are necessary to simulate these areas of abrasion or where the enamel is wearing thin allowing stronger dentine colour to filter through the enamel screen.

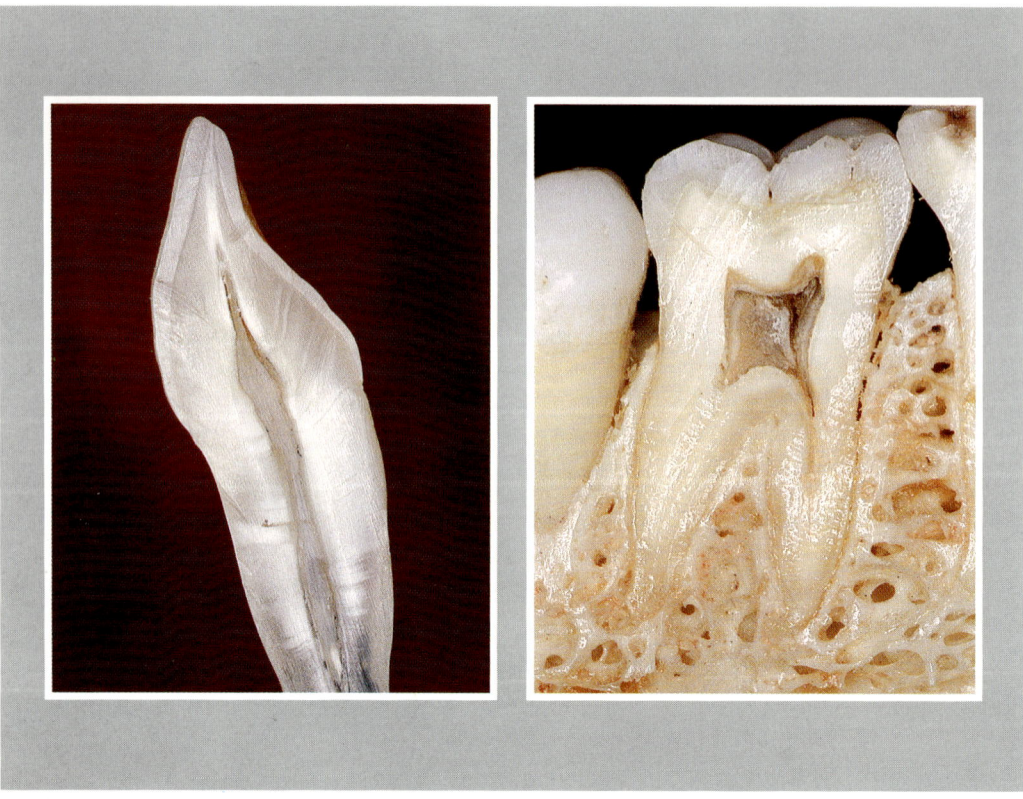

Fig 97 (left) Sectioned maxillary central. Note the thickness of the enamel and the extention of the dentine to within 0.5 mm of the incisal edge. Secondary dentine can be seen as the dense white area extending towards the incisal edge. The pulp chamber has receded thereby allowing space for the secondary dentine formation.

Fig 98 (right) Sectioned mandibular first molar here shown within the investing bone. The enamel overlay is thicker in the occlusal area when compared with anterior labial enamel thickness.

References

1. *McLean J W:* The State of the Art and its Problems in Dental Porcelains. The State of the Art 1977. Ed. Yamada H. N. Grenoble Publishing. University of Southern California.
2. *Kuwata M:* Theory and Practice for Ceramo Metal Restorations. p 35–65 Quintessence Publishing Co. 1980.
3. *Berkovitz B K, Holland G R, and Moxham B J:* A Colour Atlas and Textbook of Oral Anatomy. London: Wolfe Medical Publishing, 1968.
4. *Korson D:* The Simulation of Natural Tooth Colours in the Ceramo Metal System with Highly Chromatised Dentine Powders p 453–456 Quintessence of Dental Technology. Chicago USA No. 7 1985.
5. *Selwyn S L:* Personal communication, July, 1984.
6. *Korson D L:* Highly Chromatised Dentine Porcelains p 381–382 Perspectives in Dental Ceramics. ed. J. Preston. Quintessence Publishing Co. Chicago 1988.
7. *Yamamoto M:* Metal Ceramics p 354 Quintessence Publishing Co. Berlin. 1985.

6 Visual Building Technique

The accurate control and placement of colour characteristics has always proved difficult. The following chapter explains the visual building technique which will enable ceramists to create internal characteristics with more predictable results.

The conventional approach to building ceramic restorations is to mix porcelain powder frits with an aqueous binder to form the slurry from which the crown can be modelled. The problem for even the most competent ceramist has been the difficulty in visualizing, placing, and controlling the exact location within the tooth form of the various effects and layers such as dentine mamelons, translucent areas and white hyperplasia.

Because of an increasing awareness and co-operation between the dental researcher and the dental technician, new advances are being sought to improve many aspects of dental ceramic technology. One such advance is the introduction of organic liquid binder that is matched to the refractive index of sintered porcelain.

Refractive index

The refractive index of porcelain after the sintering process is 1.5. When a frit is not matched to the refractive index then the properties of light scattering are altered and the pre-sintered porcelain slurry will appear either more translucent or more opaque[1] than the sintered porcelain. Therefore, if a liquid with a similar refractive index can be utilized to bind the porcelain then the post-sintered state will be visualized during the building process. There are a variety of organic substances with refractive indices in the 1.5 range. These include xylene 1.49, benzene 1.5, and trichlorophenol 1.55. Oil of wintergreen has been suggested because it displays properties similar to that of the commercially available organic liquid binders, but it is too oily to be of practical use.

The introduction to the dental ceramist's armamentarium of organic liquid binders (Yamamoto[2]), which at first seemed the answer to many problems of easier control of base colour and greater accuracy for internal characterisation, has presented technical difficulties. Handling characteristics are less like the creamy consistency of water-bound porcelain slurries but are similar to uncured acrylic resin. The clumsy manipulation created for the ceramist causes difficulties in blending layers of porcelain. Therefore, so far, organic liquid binders have been of only academic use.

The visual building technique enables the dental ceramist to visualize internal modifications within the water binder build-up by the utilization of a Refractive Index

Linked (RIL) organic liquid binder[+] (fig. 99)[*].

The technique advances these binders from an academic level to a practical use.

Preparation

If porcelain frits containing organic dyes are to be used then they must be burnt off in a furnace set at 600°C for 15 minutes without vacuum so that the dyes will not influence the visualized pre-sintered colour.

It is more practical to use frits that do not contain organic dyes such as transparent and translucent powders, colour modifiers and surface stains (figs 100 and 101).

Practical application

Initially a conventional water binder build-up technique is employed. After a cut back for the enamel blend (fig 102), the colour modifications for characterisation may be added using Color Clue Liquid (fig 103). As the binder will be contaminated by water a dry brush should be employed – Color Clue Liquid is used to moisten and clean the brush. The colour characteristic can be easily visualized and the exact location and thickness judged. The viscous nature of this

---

[+] Color Cluo, Dcntal Invisions, 425-A S.E. 5th Avenue, Boynton Beach, Fl 33435 USA

[*] Care should be taken when using Color Clue Liquid as it is toxic and unpleasant side effects may result if inhaled or ingested. Avoid contact with tissues.

porcelain mixture will allow placement of the overlying enamel veneer (that will have a creamy consistency if a water binder has been used) without disturbing or merging of the internal characterisation (fig 104).

Colour verification

To be sure of the correct colour the pre-sintered sample should be placed alongside the identification tab (fig 105). For further accuracy a sample may be sintered to confirm colour and light transmission. The practice of placing a small amount of pre-sintered porcelain upon the colour identification tab to check the shade should be avoided as the natural translucency of the mixture creates a chameleon effect, and colour from the tab will transmit through to the porcelain (figs 106 and 107).

The Art of Controlling the Placement of Porcelain

Whilst it is difficult to express artistic sense it is important to try and understand the freedom of expression found by allowing shapes to occur naturally whilst adding porcelain to the build-up. Over-working of the ceramic will produce fuzzing or blurred effects whilst extensive use of a large whipping brush smooths out natural contours and creates the typical ceramic crown appearance. Examination of natural dentition under magnification will focus attention on the many small and very subtle details which many restorations lack.

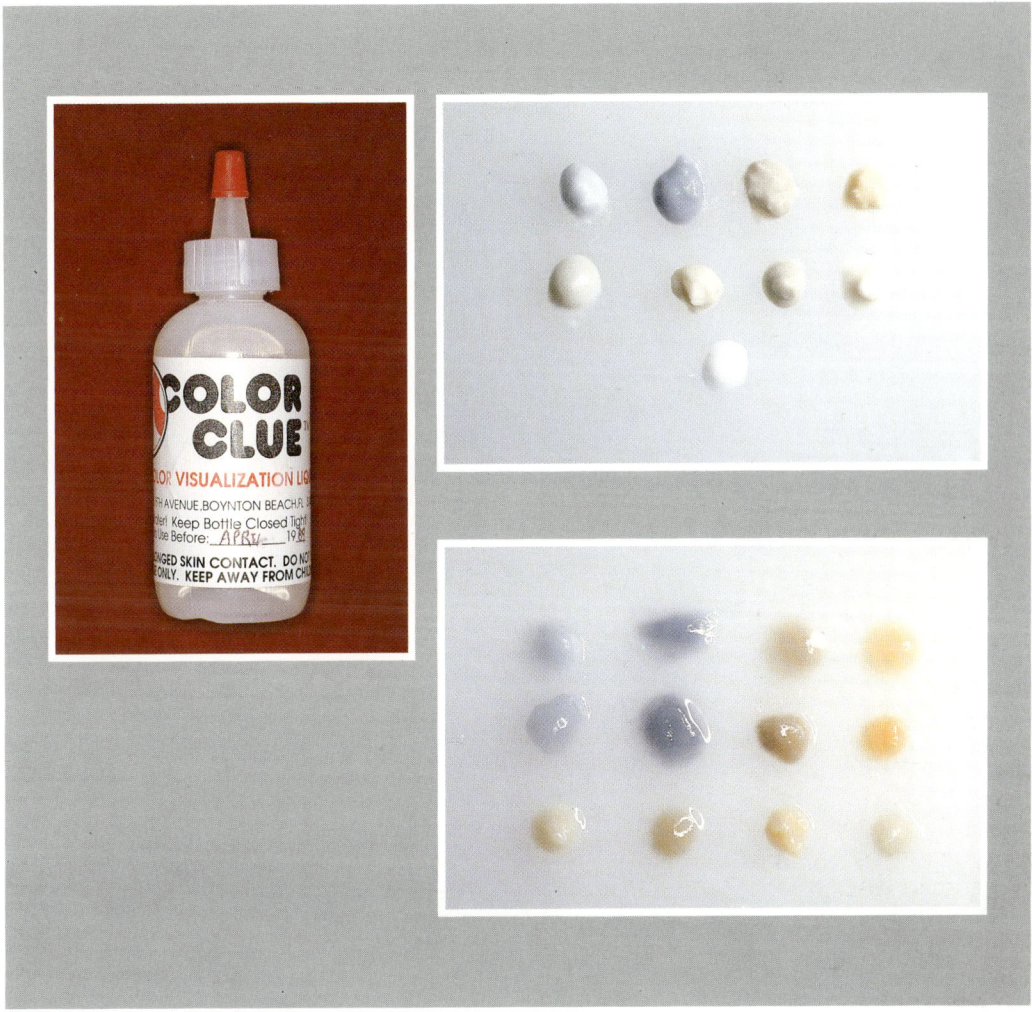

Fig 99 (left)   Visualizing liquid used to place internal characteristics.

Fig 100 (above)   Effect powders from the Creative Colour System mixed with water give no indication of the likely result after sintering.

Fig 101 (below)   The same effect powders. Top row are the same colours as the middle row, however top row were mixed with Steels Stain Liquid and are not a good match when compared with middle and lower rows mixed with Color Clue Liquid.

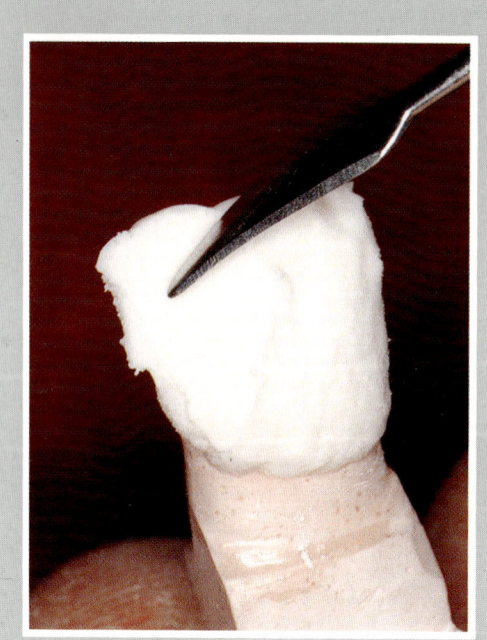

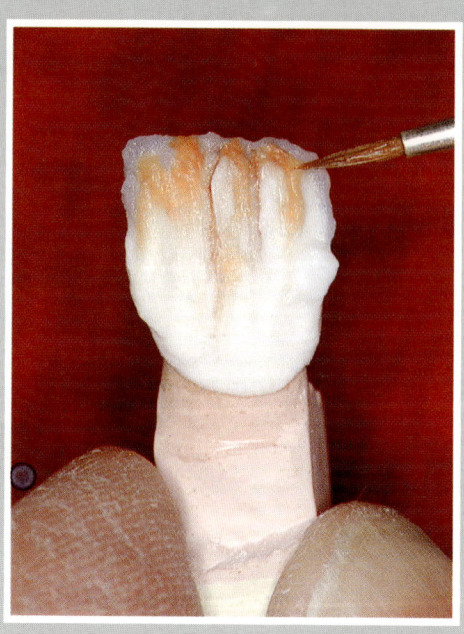

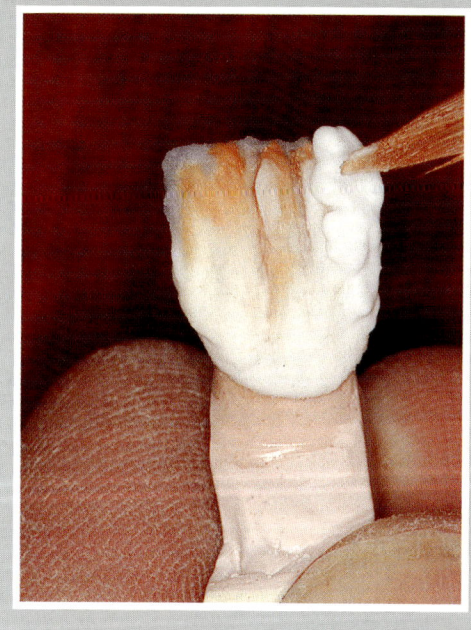

Fig. 102 (above left)   The dentine is reduced to allow room for the effect powders and the enamel overlay.

Fig 103 (above right)   The effect modifications are mixed with Color Clue Liquid and placed carefully with a small staining brush. Every colour can be accurately positioned and the post-sintered colour gauged after allowance for the diffuse effect the enamel layer will have.

Fig 104 (right)   Enamel porcelain is placed carefully over the characteristics to avoid disturbance.

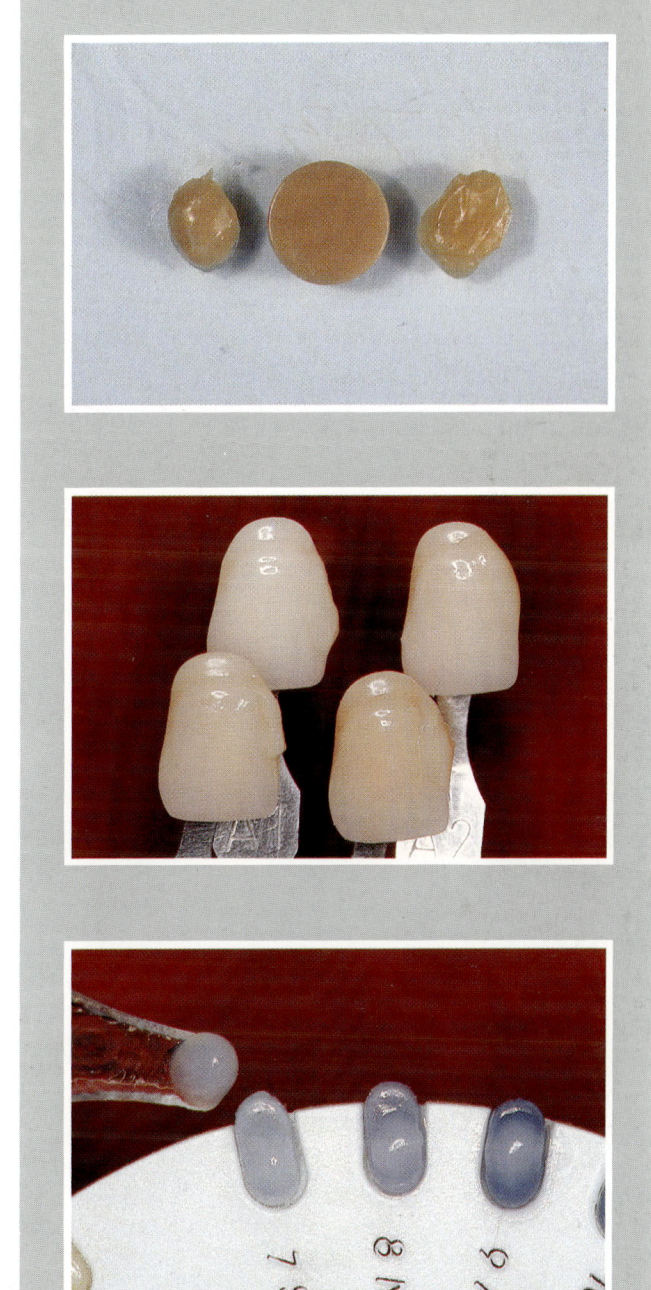

Fig 105 Samples mixed with Color Clue either side of shade disc. Left sample is good match. Right is sintered and a poor match.

Fig 106 It is incorrect to check the pre-sintered mixture by placement on the guide, as light reflected from the sample guide through the material will transmit the colour of the guide into the mixture. In this photograph CCS mamelon No. 3 has been placed upon the side of four different shade tabs, Vita A1, A2, A3, A4. As can be seen the mixture harmonises with all tabs.

Fig 107 CCS No. 7 is placed upon Nos. 7, 8, and 9. Whilst No. 7 is a good match as can be seen by the sample on the glass rod, distortion of colour on 8 and 9 is evident as the mixture is influenced by the underlying colour.

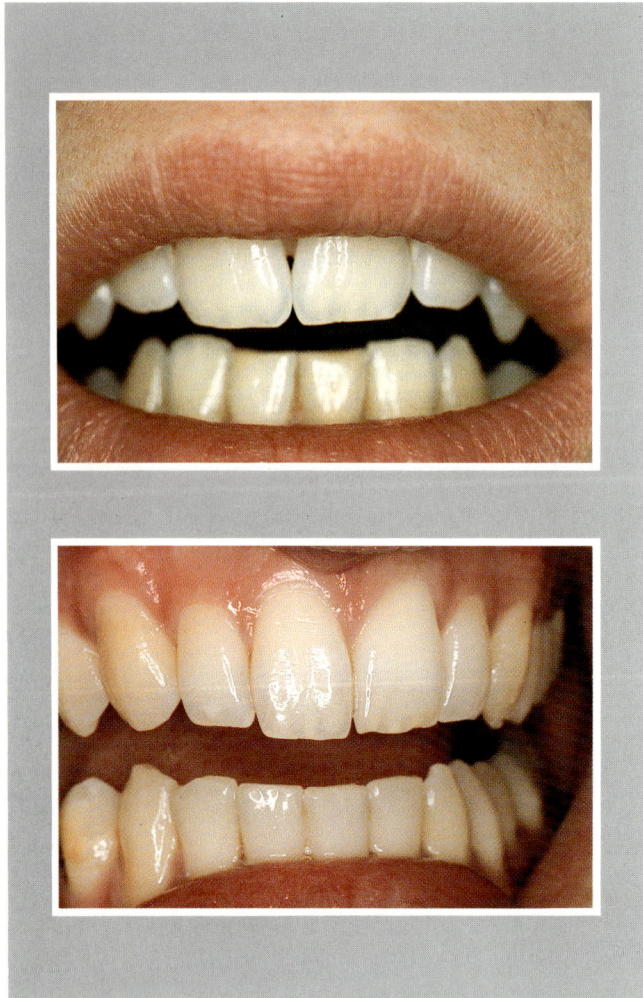

Figs 108 and 109 Natural dentition in two young patients demonstrates the incisal mamelons and blue translucent borders. The mamelons extend to the incisal edge in an irregular shape although the typical three finger formation is still evident.

6.1 Age Related Building Techniques

The character of human dentition falls into various categories and therefore one technique to build all teeth cannot be described. For this reason techniques employed to encompass a range of variants normally observed will be described using Duceram porcelain.

Young, clean, vibrant and attractive

The upper anterior central and lateral teeth in the young dentition often exhibit the typical dentine mamelons extending to approximately 1 mm short of the incisal edge, or occasionally extending to the incisal edge. The incisal edge generally appears semitransparent with a blue/grey tint, the overall effect of the enamel is opalescent (figs 108 and 109).

The typical building technique for this tooth is detailed.

Building Technique for a young dentition

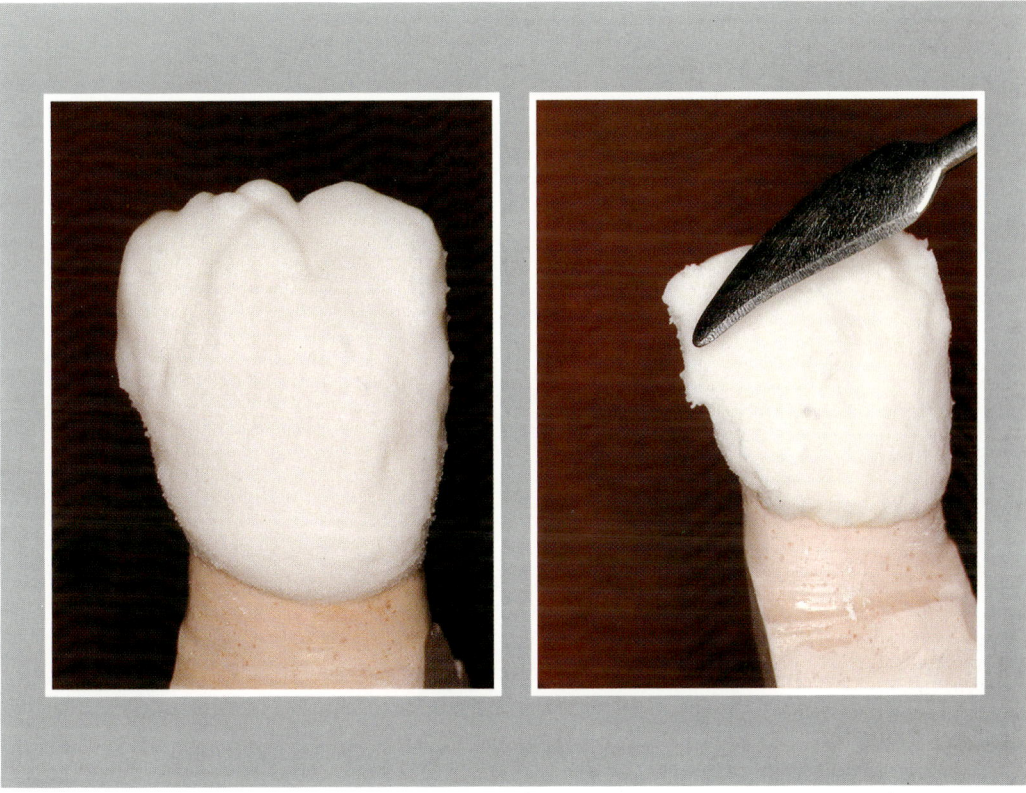

Fig 110 (left)   The diagnostic build up in dentine. This is the basis for all ceramic techniques.

Fig 111 (right)   Reduction of the dentine to allow room for modifier and enamel overlay.

Due to the clean appearance and overall white effect the layer of cervical chroma normally added beneath the basic dentine colour is omitted.

The dentine procelain build-up is commenced. Initially large increments are applied to the core until the required shape is achieved (fig 110).

The build-up in dentine is completed labially and lingually incorporating detailed anatomy, for diagnostic purposes and to control later ceramic layers.

Enamel Layer Cut Back
Cut back the labial face extending in a gentle bevel to the cervical third and in a gentle curve mesio-distally (fig 111). **This is the basic cut back technique employed throughout.**

In cases where a translucent blue incisal border is indicated then dentine reduction is cut into the incisal edge. This technique is only used in instances where maximum light transmission through the incisal edge is required (figs 112 to 117).

Incisal blue is placed carefully by using Color Clue Liquid. This will prevent the colour characteristics merging with the dentine build-up and losing distinction (fig 118).

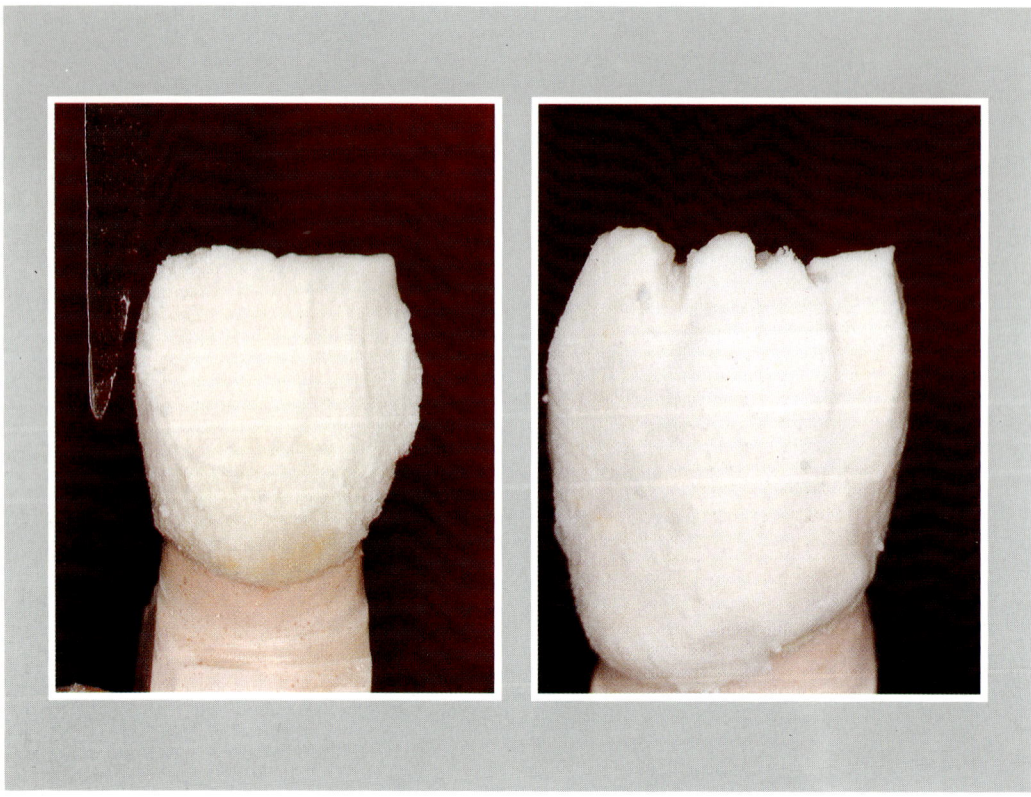

Fig 112 (left) Reduction of the mesial and distal walls to allow the placement of blue modifier.

Fig 113 (right) Creating a natural incisal dentine opacity, as in examples of natural dentition Fig. 108 and 109. The incisal edge is broken and made irregular.

Relationship between the approximate length of final build-up and the level of dentine cut back, allowing for sintering contraction

Figs 114 and 115 (page 71, above) Dentine reduction Type A, to allow space for a translucent incisal border.

Figs 116 and 117 (below) Dentine reduction Type B, for the typical building technique where dentine is carried to within 1 mm of the incisal edge when less translucency is required.

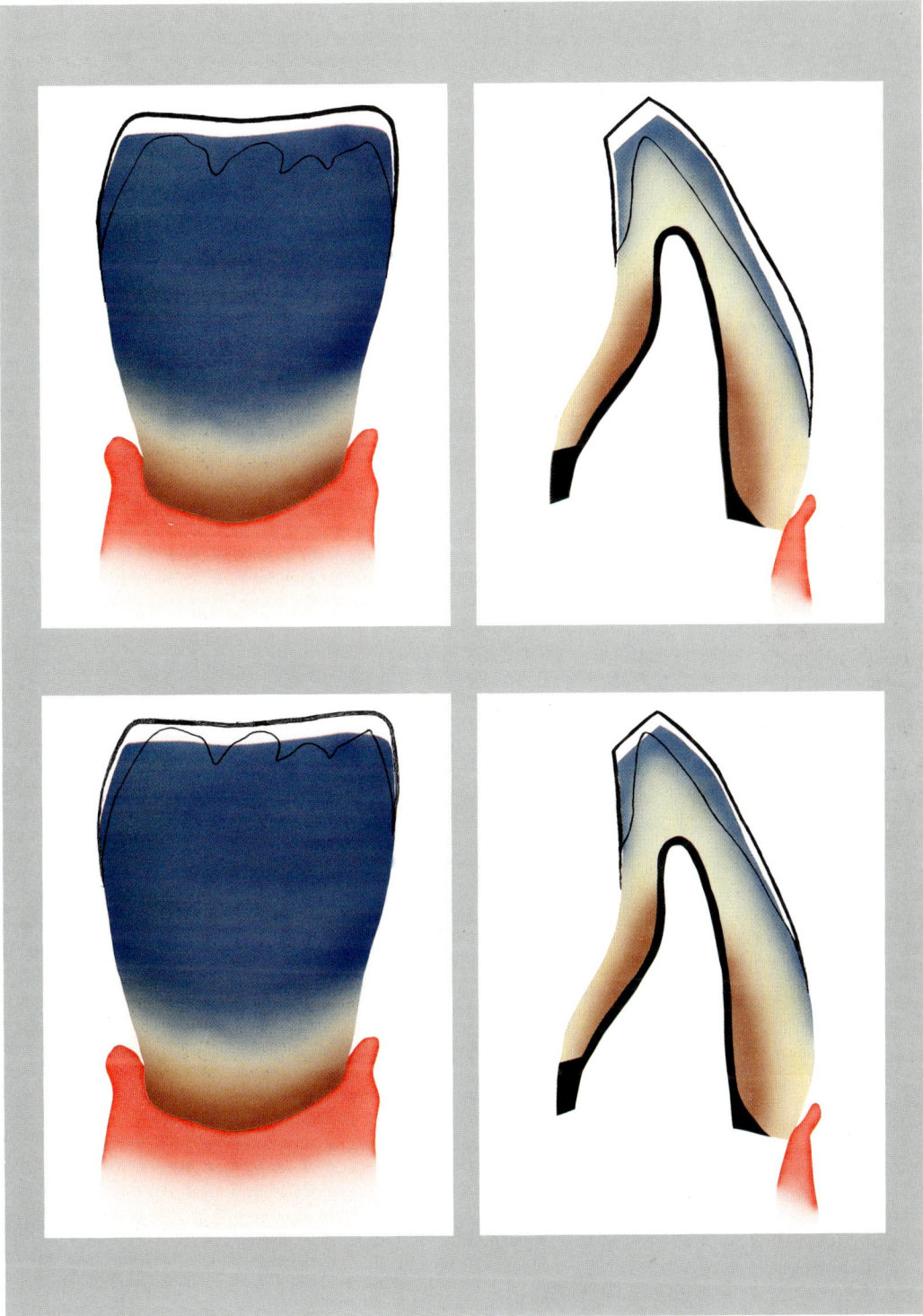

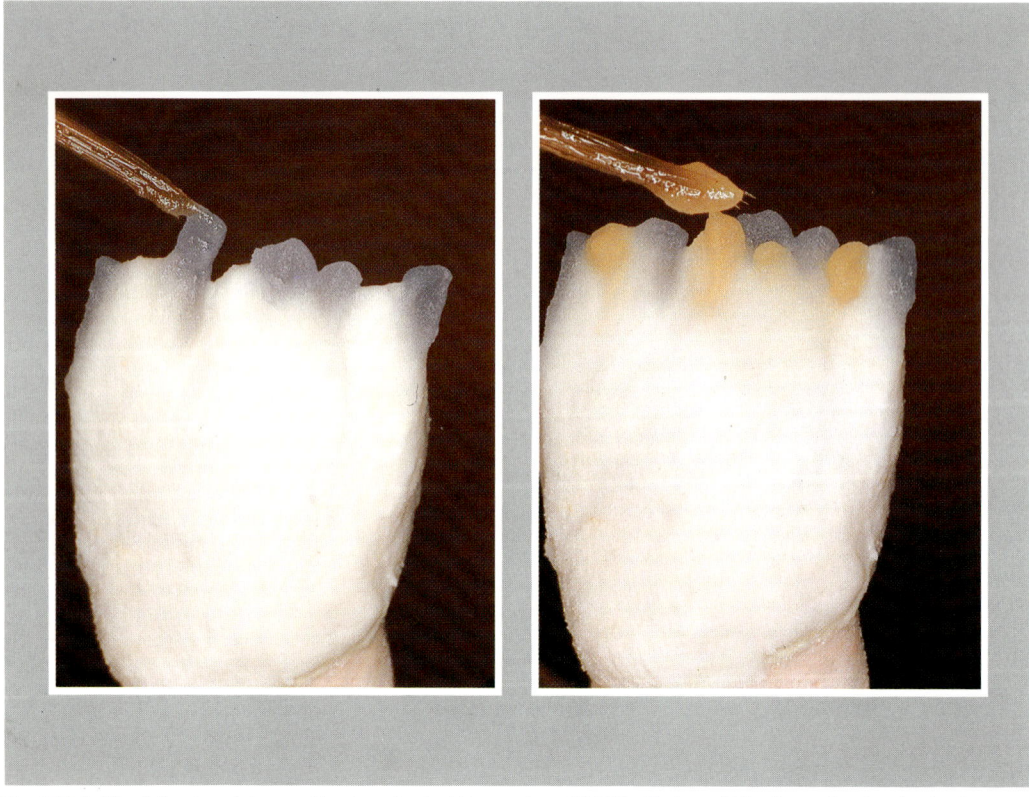

Fig. 118 (left)   A fine brush is used to place incisal blue colour CCS No. 7 at or a little above the dentine build-up to create additional translucency. (Dentine Reduction Type A)

Fig 119 (right)   Mamelon colour CCS No. 3 is placed into the correct position according to shade instructions or photograph. (Note: Mamelon colour has been intensified for photographic clarity.)

Care should be taken not to place too much blue in this region or to smudge the detail as this will create an unnatural blue/grey cast through the enamel.

Mamelon colour is also placed into the correct position (fig 119). The use of photographs to aid the correct positioning for these effects proves an invaluable aid (see figs 24 and 25).

The Enamel Layer
Returning to water-based porcelain the enamel layer is placed over the colour characteristics and, in this case, a multiple horizontal band technique is employed. Various frits, ranging from translucent clear through white and grey enamels to translucent opalescent, are employed throughout the building technique. This will achieve various effects by allowing the influence from the underlying dentine to show through or by creating whiter areas of enamel with the use of translucent opalescent. The effect of polishing the finished ceramic adds a quality to translucent clear which allows more light penetration.

For these reasons the building programme for the enamel layer serves as a guide to useful technique but may be varied according to the desired effect.

The first layer of translucent clear is carefully placed at the incisal border avoiding

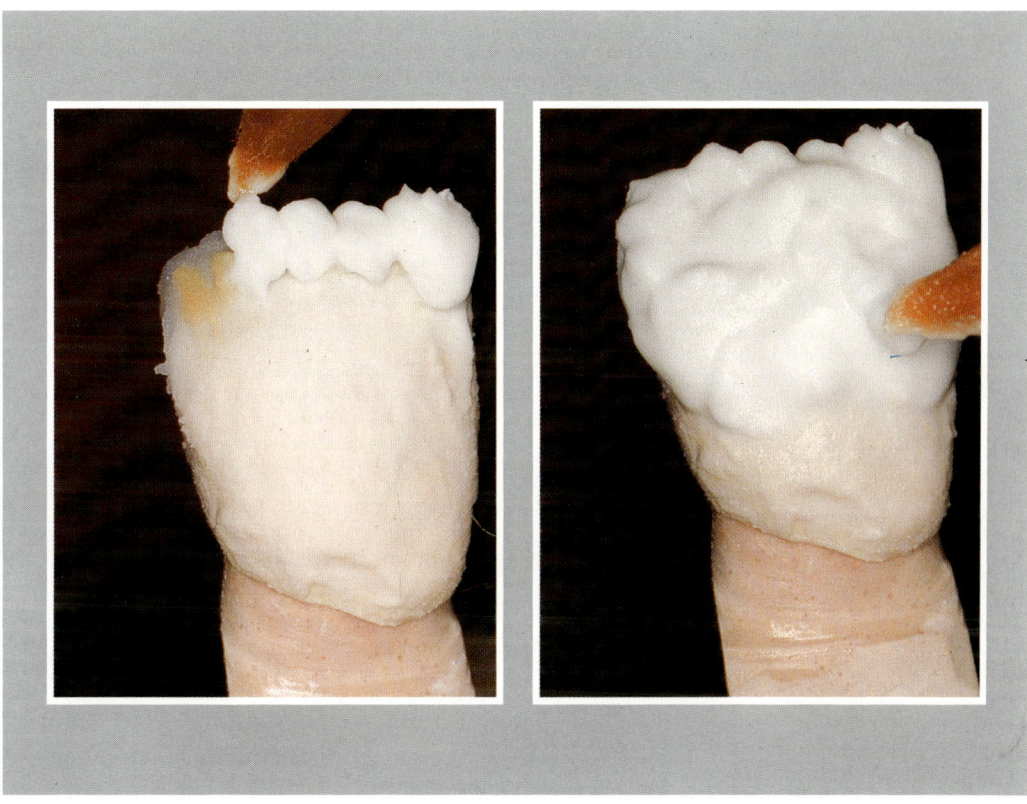

Fig 120 (left)   Example of placement of characteristics in Dentine Reduction Type B. Translucent clear is used as the first layer of enamel in both Type A and B Reduction.

Fig 121 (right)   S. 57 is used as the next layer of enamel to be placed at the middle third of the tooth. This will simulate the opalescent enamel of young dentition.

disturbing the characteristics (fig 120). This is to allow the colours built at the incisal to filter through and to create more grey translucency in this area, extending beyond the incisal edge to compensate for sintering shrinkage.

The second horizontal band is placed at the middle third of the tooth. In this example S57 is used as it is a whitish enamel intended for Al-Bl and simulates the appearance of the young tooth with opalescent enamel (fig. 121).

The third band placed is a translucent opalescent at the cervical third to allow some enamel influence in this region. As this layer is likely to be thin translucent

opalescent will have more effect than S57 enamel. In addition the white opalescent quality adds vitality to the area (figs 122 and 123).

Middle-aged, individual, with vitality

As with other aspects of human anatomy the aging process varies between individuals, with the middle-aged bridging the gap between youth and the elderly. Their teeth reflect this.

The dentition in the middle-aged has the greatest variation in character, ranging from healthy youthful vitality to teeth with

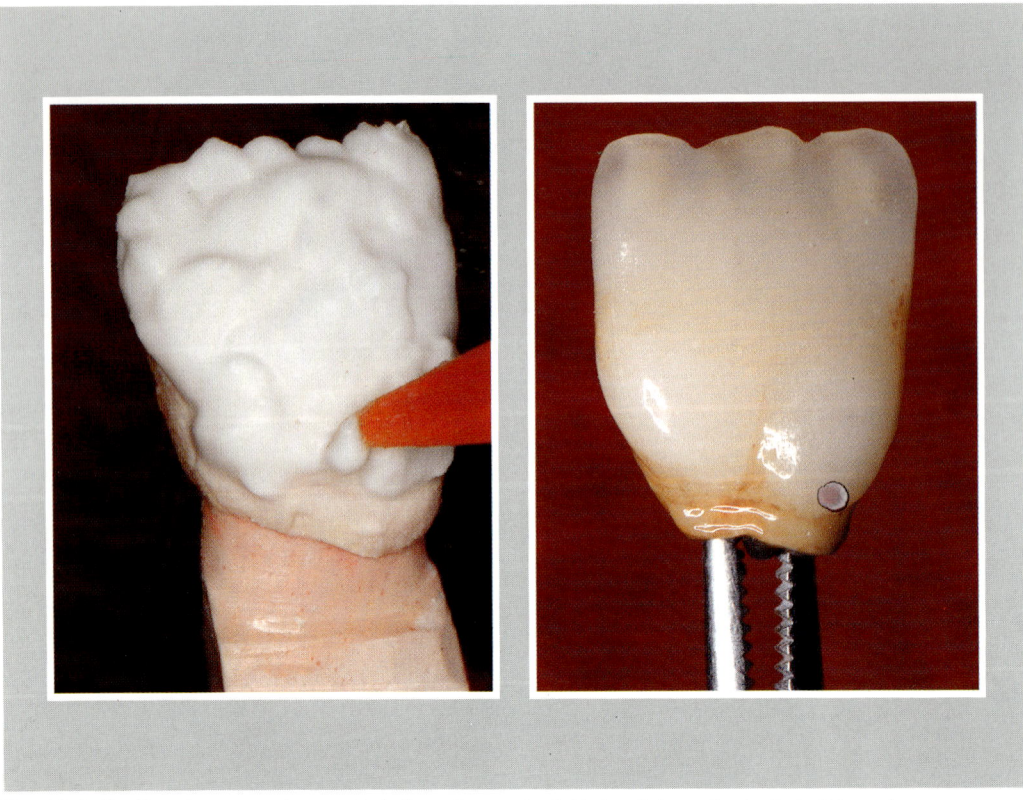

Fig 122 (left)   Translucent opalescent is built at the cervical third to lighten the tooth in this region.

Fig 123 (right)   Completed tooth of the typical young dentition with incisal blue translucent border, mamelon effects and opalescence in the cervical third (Dentine Reduction Type A).

exposed necks, small pits, darker colour and enamel with an opalescent quality shining through a translucent overlay.

The following description is of a typical "middle-aged tooth".

Slightly darker in overall colour, the dentine mamelons have been replaced by secondary dentine which is less pronounced, appearing as a faint horizontal yellow/orange band across the incisal third. The enamel overlay displays an opalescence shining through an almost transparent overlay. A small degree of tissue recession has exposed the root surface.

Surface characteristics are becoming smooth and polished, allowing light to penetrate the translucent overlay through to the opalescent enamel and into the dentine which is then reflected back to the observer's eye. The overall effect is of a rich vital colour beneath a translucent opalescent enamel.

The typical building technique for this tooth is detailed.

To create additional colour within the crown, High Chroma Dentine is laid mesially, distally and just extending onto the face of the tooth (fig 124).

The dentine build-up is made to full contour extending beyond the incisal edge to compensate for sintering shrinkage (Dentine Reduction Type B). This is normal prac-

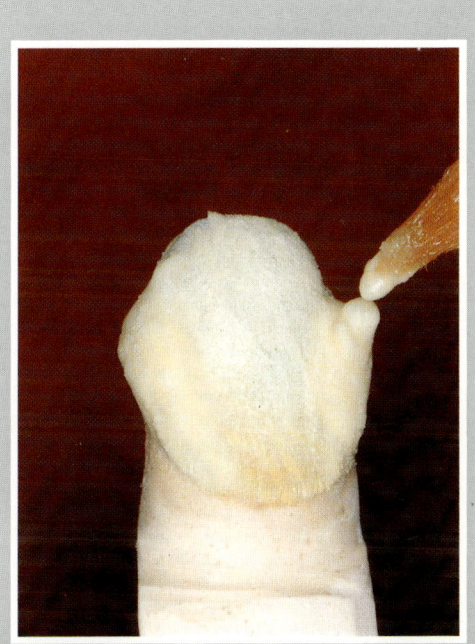

Building Technique for the middle-aged dentition

Fig 124 (left)   The opaque has been modified to harmonise with the final colour of the crown, particularly at the cervical third. High Chroma Dentine is placed around the marginal area and extended up the proximal walls. In this case the mixture is for Vita A3, and therefore is DA3 and CCS No. 22 1:1 (refer to Table 5 page 59)

Fig 125 (below left)   Dentine porcelain DA3 is built to the tooth shape with extension incisally, to allow for sintering shrinkage.

Fig 126 (below right)   After cutting away the mesial and distal incisal corner CCS No. 7 blue is placed into position.

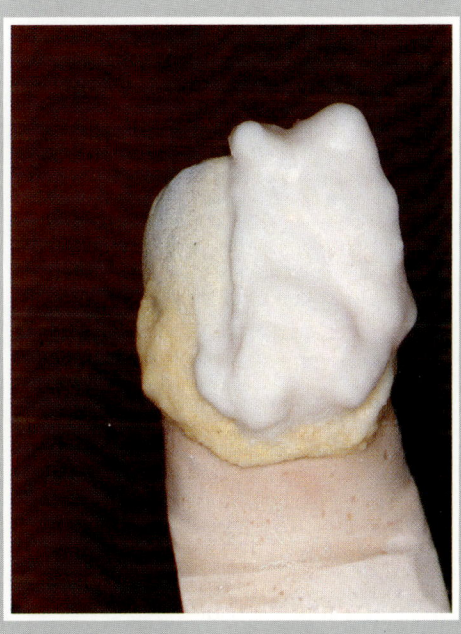

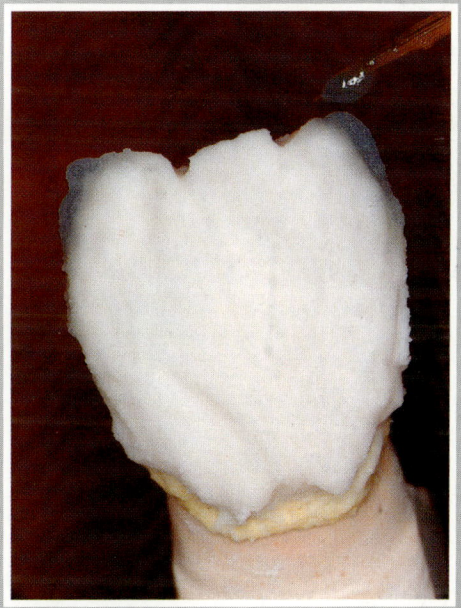

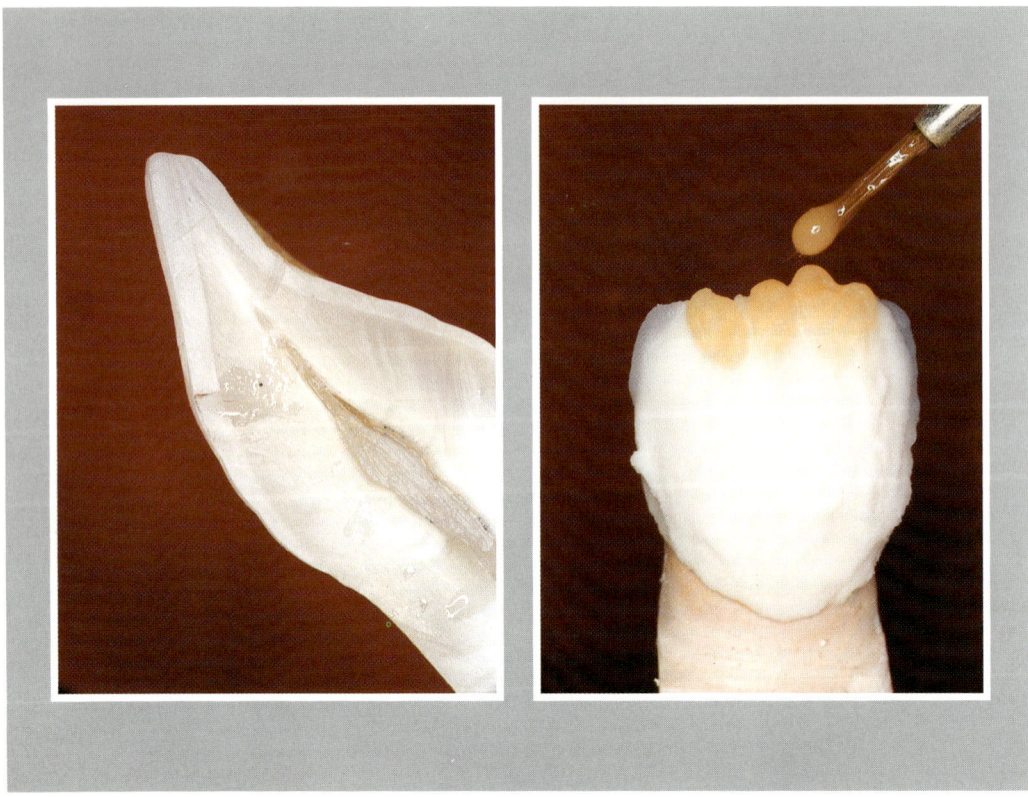

Fig 127 (left)   Cross-section of natural maxillary central shows the dentine and secondary dentine extending almost to the incisal edge. This is how the dentine is built within the crown. By extending the dentine incisally to compensate for sintering shrinkage and reducing it for enamel both lingually and labially a similar relationship will exist (see also figs 114 to 117).

Fig 128 (right)   Secondary dentine formation using mamelon colour CCS No. 4 is placed in a continuous but irregular band of colour across the incisal region (Note: Mamolon colour has been intensified for photographic clarity.)

Figs 129 and 130 (page 77, above)   Enamel porcelain S58 is placed over the entire face of the tooth.

Fig 131 (below left)   Enamel porcelain is brushed away to almost expose the characteristics and translucent clear is built over. This is to create enamel opalescence showing from within a translucent tooth.

Fig 132 (below right)   Completed crown for the middle-aged dentition demonstrating all the characteristics. The areas of blue incisal and secondary dentine can be seen through the enamel. A root has been developed. Characteristic morphology is important to prevent an unnatural appearance in multiple units.

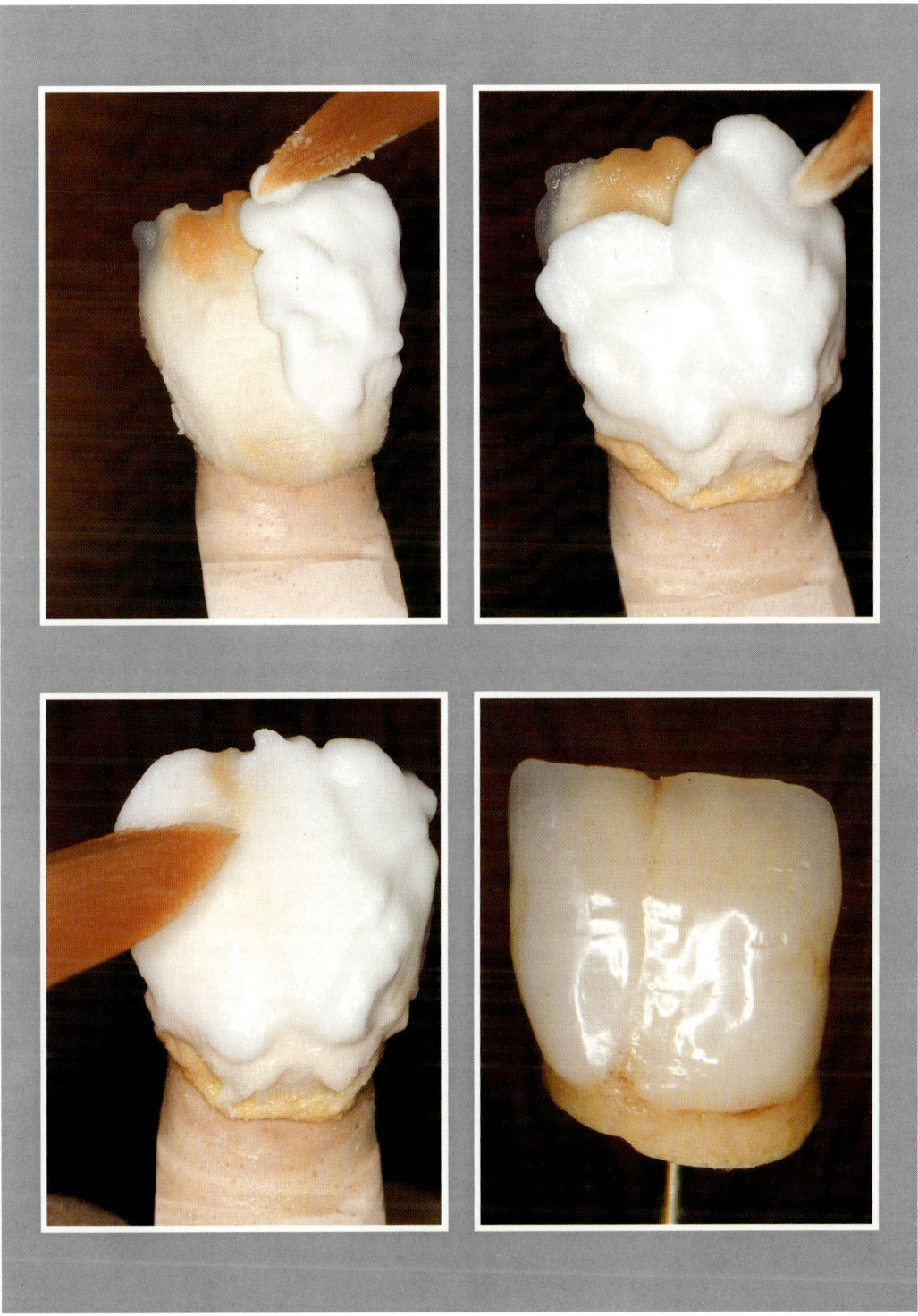

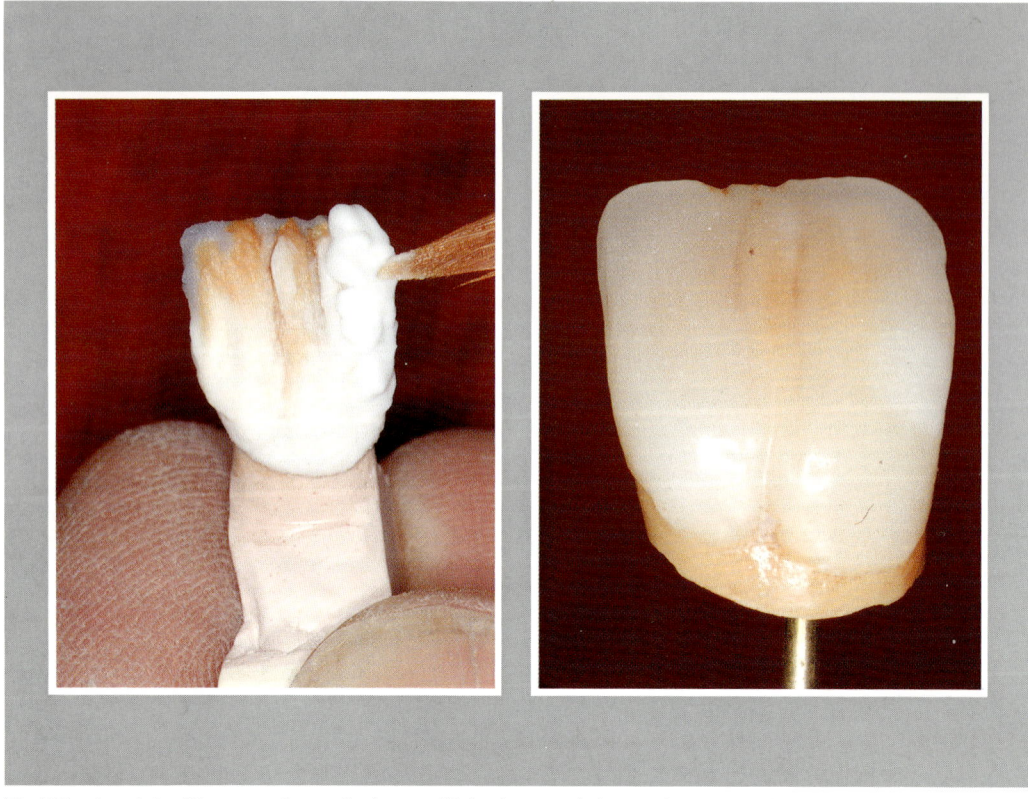

Fig 133 Aged dentition sometimes displays multiple characteristics such as secondary dentine, incisal blue and dark yellow or brown straining.
All these characteristics are placed in the build-up using Color Clue Liquid. Intense yellow and brown hues are made by adding surface stains to Creative Colour System dentines and therefore only a small amount of stain is placed within the build up. This is important as surface stains have a tendency to discolour, becoming more intense than intended when they are sintered. Enamel layers are built over the internal characteristics.

Fig 134 The completed crown for the aged dentition.

Figs 135 to 143 (page 79)
Fig 135 Color Clue Liquid has the ability to generate a close to true colour for the ceramic, providing the build-up is moist. The colour remains accurate, here seen corresponding to CCS No. 7 Incisal Blue.

Fig 136 Characteristic corresponds to CCS No. 3 Mamelon.

Fig 137 The completed crown shows the internal mamelon colour still remains true to the colour wheel.

Fig 138 Blue at the incisal edge.

Figs 139 and 140 The root area.

Fig 141 to 143 Comparison of the three samples in the age groupings, young, middle-aged and aged.

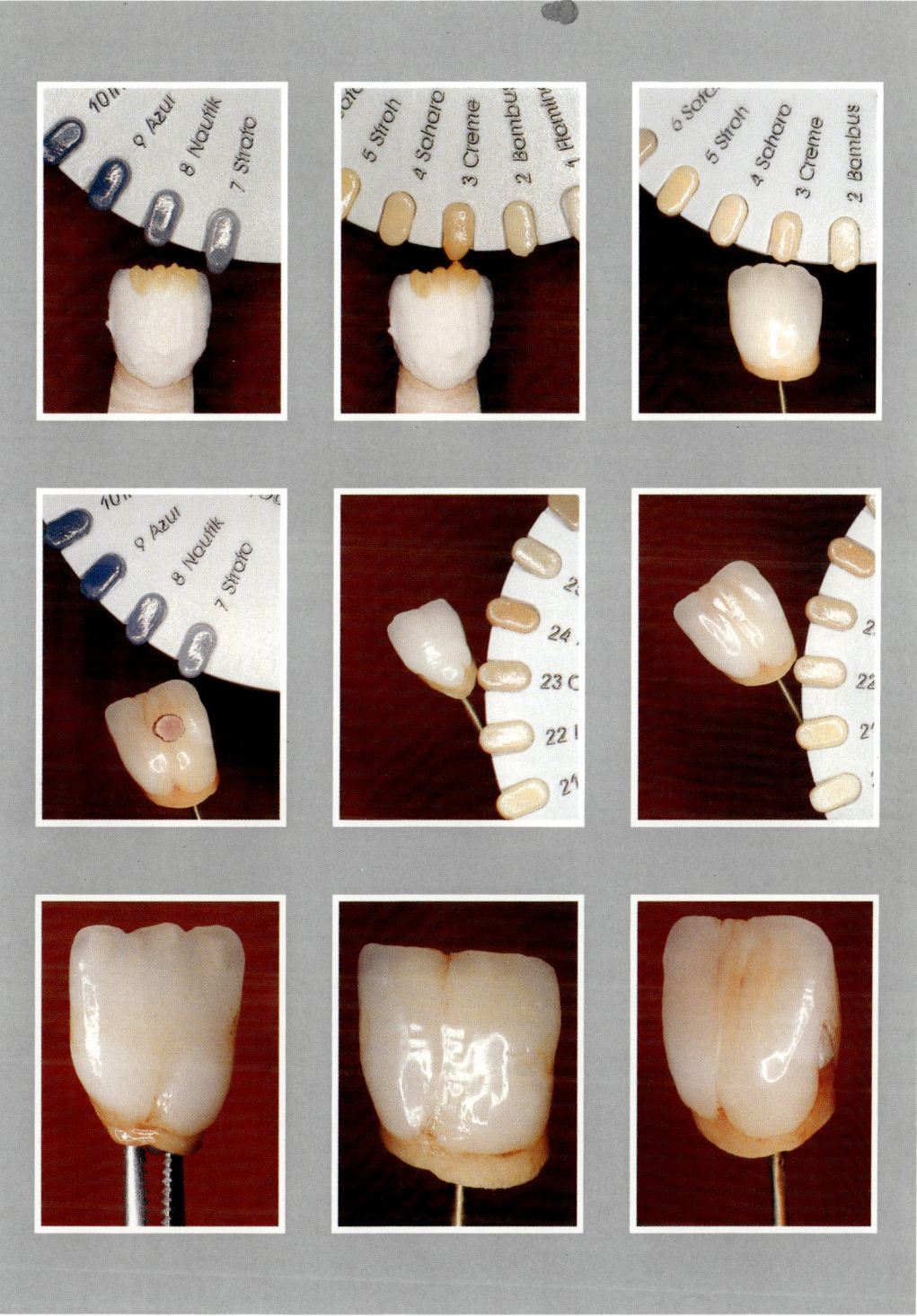

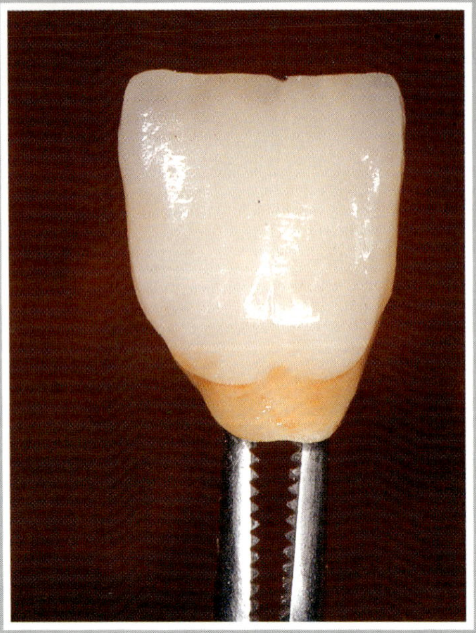

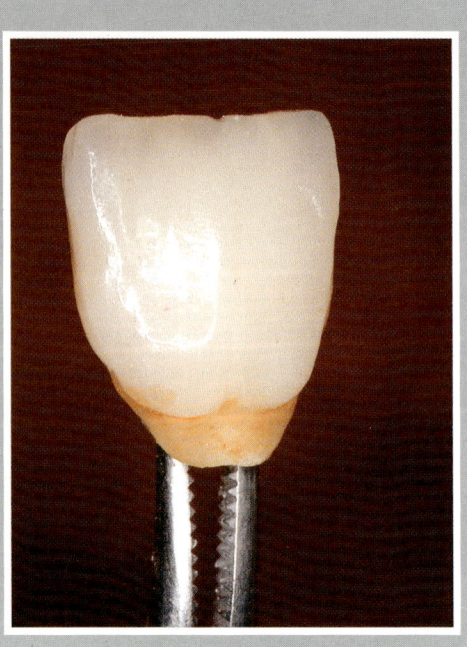

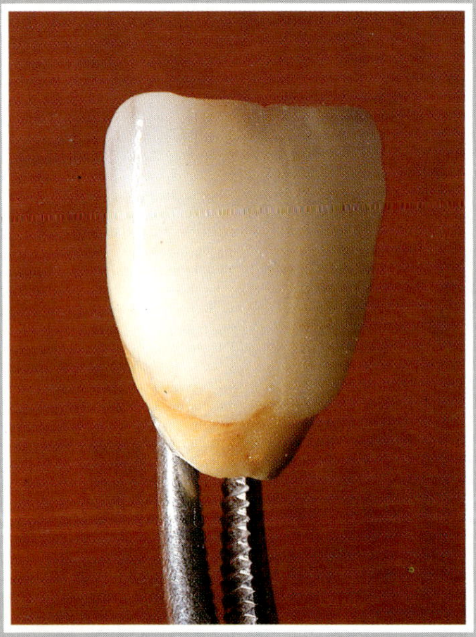

Fig 144 (above left) Porcelain crown with built in pale white enamel crack. As can be seen the crack line is invisible from this view.

Figs 145 and 146 As the tooth rotates and the angle of view is from a lateral position the crack becomes more obvious.

tice in all cases except in the situation where a translucent halo is present, as with the preceding paragraphs relating to young teeth (figs 125 and 126; see also figs 114 to 117).

When comparing a natural tooth (fig 127) it is evident that the dentine extends almost to the incisal edge and it is to simulate this situation that the crown is built in the same way. Therefore, after the cut back for the enamel labially and also lingually, a thin wedge of dentine is left extending almost to the incisal edge. This also prevents the typical grey incisal hue with which many ceramic restorations are plagued.

The incisal no longer displays the three finger mamelon effect. Instead secondary dentine influences the colour which becomes yellow and darker with the aging process. Ducera CCS No. 4 is laid in an irregular fashion across this region using Color Clue Liquid; this will appear as a faint band of colour across the incisal third (fig 128).

The Enamel Layer
To simulate a deep opalescence from within a translucent overlay, the enamel is built as two layers. The first should be pale white in colour (such as S58) and is applied by flowing over almost the entire face of the crown, stopping just short of the cervical margin and taking care to avoid disturbing any internal characterisation such as the secondary dentine. This opalescent enamel layer should be thinned by blending back to almost expose the internal characterisation. The second layer is flowed over, using translucent clear thereby creating the effect of a translucent overlay. Once again this will become much more effective following surface polishing techniques after glazing (figs 129 to 131).

Teeth for the elderly – colourful with character

Due to the wearing process teeth for the aged have thin polished enamel and there-fore more dentine colour is reflected back to the observer's eye. Incisal edges are likely to be worn flat and areas of abrasion are often observed on the incisal edge. In addition slight incisal chipping may occur and gingival recession will expose tooth roots which are likely to have stained to dark colours. Discoloured enamel cracks and pits are common.

To generate more chroma at the cervical third CCS root dentine of the appropriate colour, in this case No. 23, is applied.

The dentine is built and the reduction for enamel is described under the section for Middle-aged teeth.

Areas of discolouration emanating from the dentine may be incorporated at this stage. Brown, orange-brown or yellow are common and the exact colours can be verified with a visualising liquid (fig 133).

The Enamel Layer
Because in most older people the enamel layer has become more translucent, a water-based mixture of translucent clear with 10% dentine is laid over the incisal and body portion of the tooth face as the enamel overlay. Cervical opalescence has been incorporated with the use of translucent opalescent (fig 134).

6.2 Additional Tooth Characteristics

The inclusion and duplication of the various individual characteristics commonly occurring in normal dentition will enhance aesthetic results and create harmony, allowing artificial teeth to blend with natural dentition. It is the simulation of pertinent individual characteristics which prevent the restoration appearing monochromatic, uniform and artificial.

Enamel Cracks

The duplication of enamel cracks in ceramics requires an understanding by the

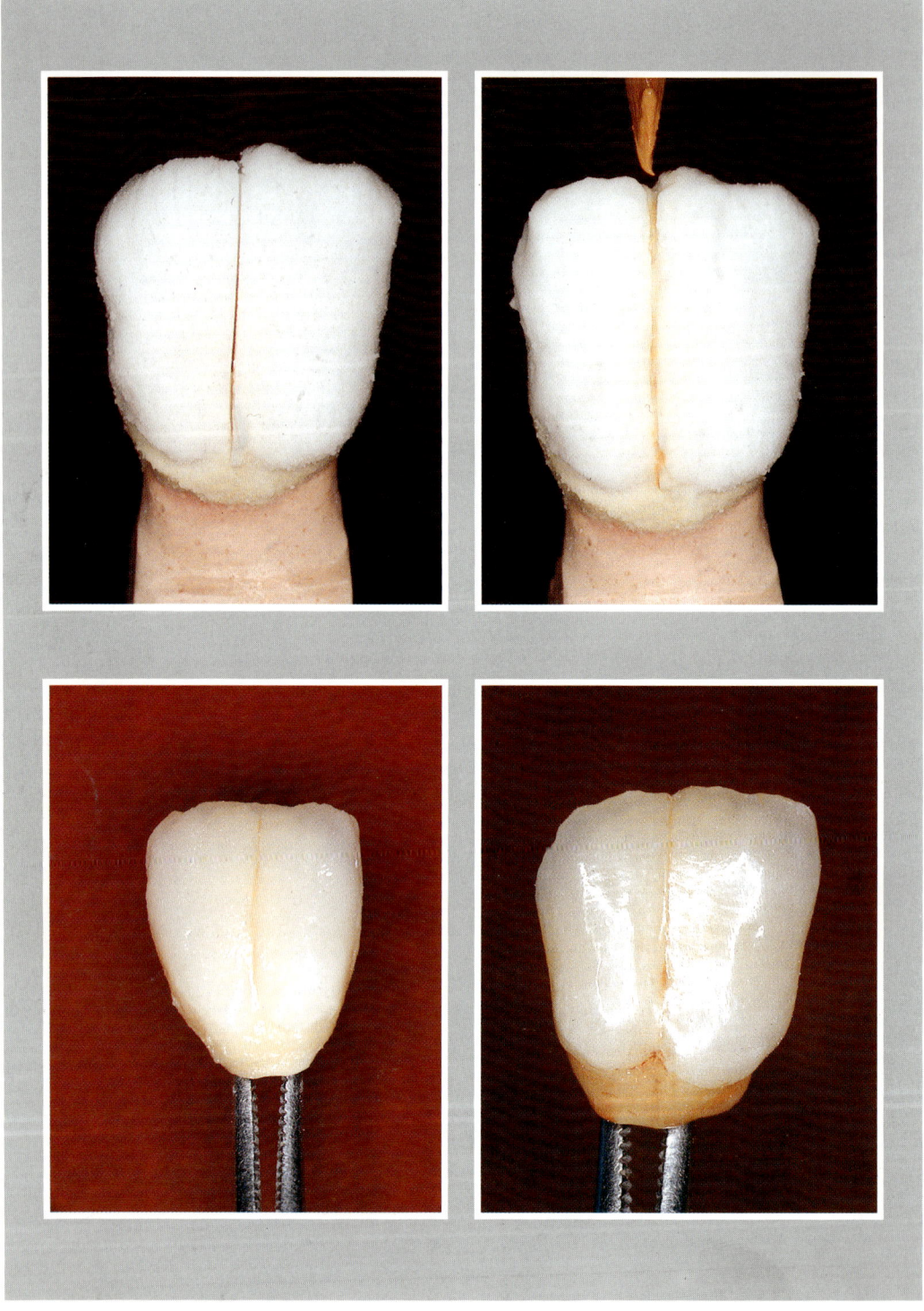

Building Technique to produce fine vertical crack lines

Figs 147 to 150 (page 82) In this case (type 2) a fine orange crack which is just becoming open at the surface.
Fig 147 All building processes are carried through until only the crack characteristic is required. A thin blade is used to cut a fine crack into the damp build-up.

Fig 148 Using a No. 8 brush, a weak solution of orange surface stain material is lightly touched to the crack. If the build-up is sufficiently moist the surface stain will be drawn quickly into the cut by capillary action.

Fig 149 Crown after sintering.

Fig 150 Completed crown following further corrective firings for the crown contour.

ceramist of exactly which type is required and the precise technique necessary for reproduction.

The formation of stress cracks within the tooth enamel fall into five categories.

1. Fine enamel cracks which appear as a straight vertical line, pale cream to yellow in colour, invisible when the line of view is straight and only becoming visible from a lateral view.

Often the angle of the crack to the labial face is close to 90°. In this situation face observation focuses only the edge of the crack, therefore the small crack width is difficult to see. As the observer moves to view from a lateral position the angle of view is altered and the crack will be more obvious.

The more oblique the angle of view, the more visible the crack will become. Observation of the crack is only possible because of a minute air space which interrupts the passage of light through the enamel. The crack remains unstained, i. e. pale cream to yellow, because at this stage it is closed at the enamel surface (figs. 144 to 146).

2. Middle-aged dentition often exhibits fine straight cracks in the enamel which are just becoming open to the surface. These cracks are light orange in colour with low intensity and therefore only just visible to the naked eye.

3. As the dentition ages the crack widens and the ingress of oral fluids and bacteria stain the crack to a dark brown colour.

Technique for crack types 1, 2 and 3

Complete the build-up and, ensuring that the porcelain is damp, make a fine cut where the crack is required. If a razor blade is used then this must be thinned to 0.1 mm evenly across the width of the blade. Damp the porcelain until it appears slightly moist and at this stage run a thin water-based slurry of surface stain of the correct colour into the crack. Capilliary action will draw the stain deep into the cut.

It is important to use a No. 8 size brush and not a fine stain brush as sufficient moisture must be retained in the bristles to allow a reservoir of water to be available for the capillary action to draw the water from the brush into the crack (figs 147 to 150).

4. Occasionally faults within the enamel appear as a multitude of curved cracks running through the enamel at a shallow angle to the tooth surface, i. e. less than 90°. These will be observed more easily from a straight view due to the oblique angle of the crack to the observer's eye.

Technique for crack type 4

These are best built using the lateral segmental building technique.[3,4] The enamel layer is built in vertical strips across the face of the tooth and each segment has a well defined edge approximately 90° to the labial face. Since the line to be painted

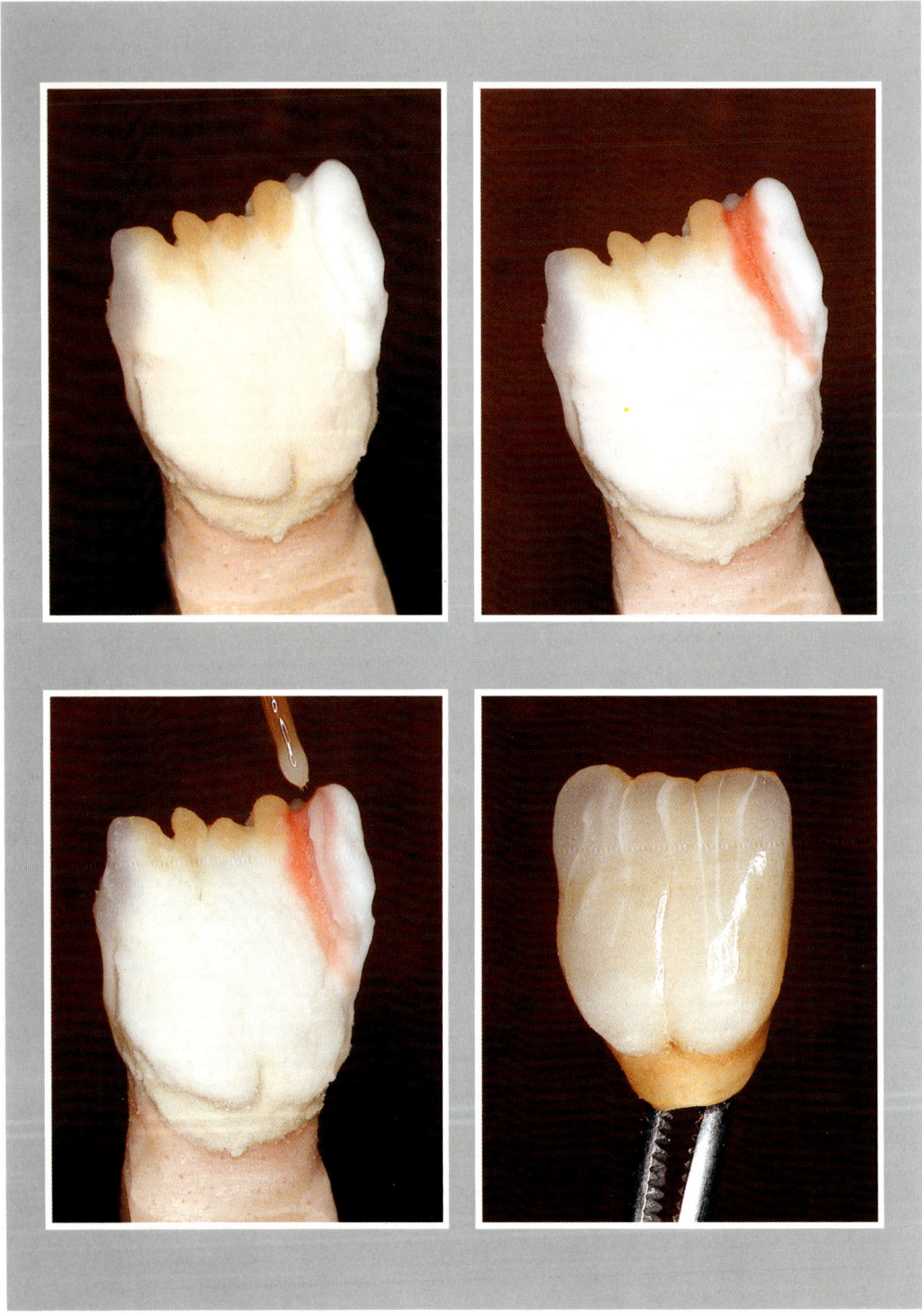

Building technique to produce multiple curved cracks within the enamel

Figs 151 to 154 (page 84)

Fig 151   After internal characteristics are placed the enamel wall is developed with a well defined and contoured wall emanating from the crown face at an angle of 90°.

Fig 152   Because the line is to be white and the enamel wall is also white, a vegetable dye is used to colour the wall in order that the painted line will be seen at this stage.

Fig 153   Ducera Cargo powder is used to make the white line as this is pale white in colour, unlike modifiers or stain which are too intense. The Cargo powder is mixed with Color Clue Liquid. In this way the powder will not diffuse into the dentine. Further lines may be created by continuing the technique across the labial face of the tooth.

Fig 154   Completed crown with a multitude of curved crack lines. This appearance cannot be simulated with surface staining techniques.

against this wall is to be pale white and the enamel is also white, it is necessary to shade the area with a dark vegetable dye in order that the white line can be seen as it is applied. Against this edge is laid the white line, Cargo powder with Color Clue Liquid as the carrier medium may be used without additional colourants for a pale white line. Mixing a little Vita* 702 surface stain with Ducera Cargo powder will provide a pale yellow line.

Color Clue Liquid is preferred to water for two reasons. First so that an approximation of the colour may be seen and second to prevent the line seeping into the build up, which is a problem if water is used as the carrier medium. Additional lines are built as required placing a thin strip of enamel or enamel and clear mixture between each line. Should a curved appearance be required it is possible to push and distort the build-up to the shape required for the lines.[4]

* Vita Zahnfabrik, D-7880 Bad Säckingen, Postfach 1338, W. Germany.

However this is only practical for one or two cracks; if many more are required then these need to be built to the contour required (figs 151 to 154).

5. The final category of crack is the diffused pale white line laying within the enamel. Unlike a fine enamel crack, this appears much thicker.

Technique for the Diffused Line

The diffused line should be laid onto a shallow cut back within the enamel layer at a depth from the surface of approximately 0.2 mm. Cargo powder is mixed with water to allow the mixture to be diffused. Using a fine stain brush, a thin slurry is run onto the moist build-up (figs 155 to 157).

Dentine Mamelons

– see section Age Related Building Techniques – Young, clean, vibrant and attractive.

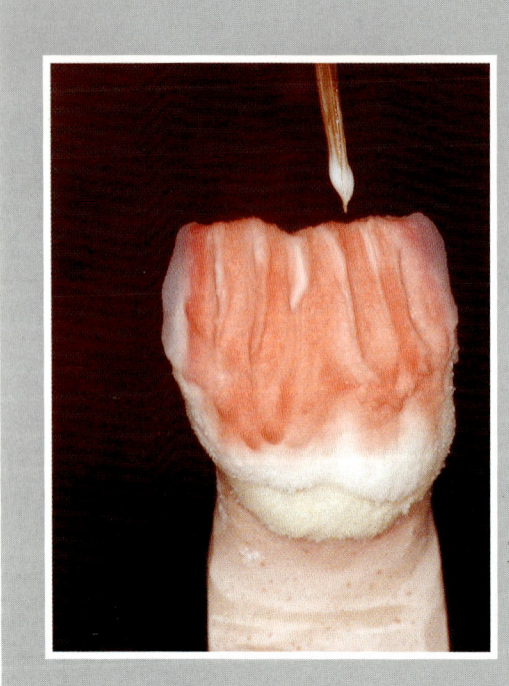

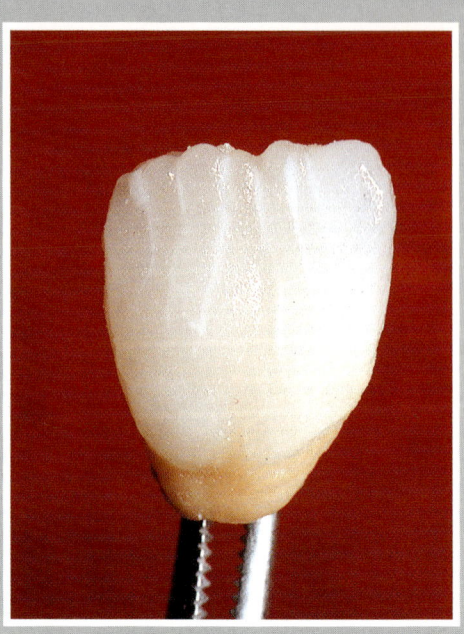

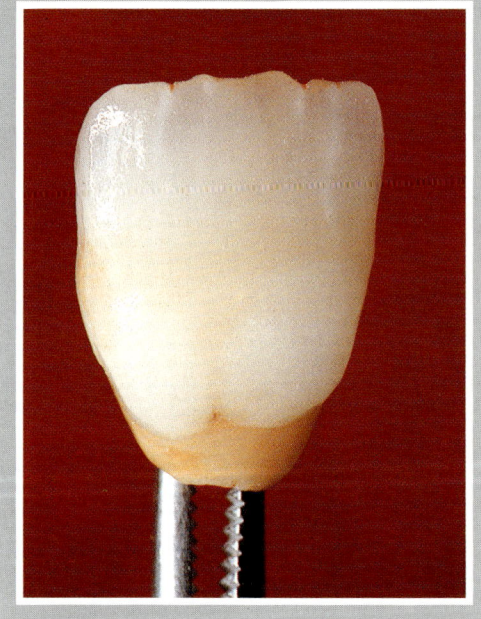

Fig 155 (above)   Technique to duplicate diffused white lines appearing beneath the enamel. Shallow cut back within the enamel layer is coloured with vegetable dye so that Ducera Cargo powder may be seen when painted onto the build-up. As the lines are to be diffused the powder is mixed with water. Slight refinement with a fine brush may be necessary after placement of the lines.

Fig 156 (above right)   Crown as it appears after sintering.

Fig 157 (right)   Lines were considered over-emphasised, therefore crown was completed after reduction of excess white by grinding and an addition of enamel porcelain.

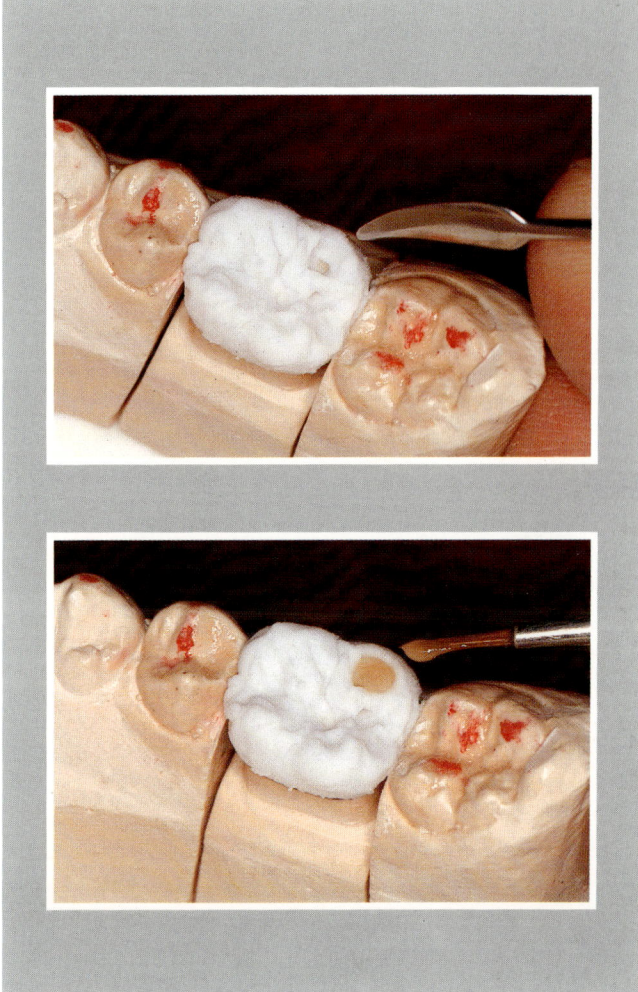

Fig 158 Abrasion lesions may be simulated by completing the build-up, then removing enamel in the region of the lesion ensuring a deep, well-defined cavity.

Fig 159 Replace with chromatised dentine in this case CCS No. 16. Apricot.

Enamel Abrasion with Stained Dentine

Incisal edges or cusp tips which suffer enamel abrasion, exposing dentine which becomes stained, may be simulated by removing enamel from the completed build-up and replacing with the correct colour of chromatised dentine (figs 158 and 159).

Enamel Surface Pits

Often discoloured pits are present in the natural dentition and, whilst most patients do not wish these to be included in the restorative work, occasionally the need arises to simulate this character to blend with the surrounding dentition. Care should be taken to select the correct colour and to avoid over-emphasizing the effect.

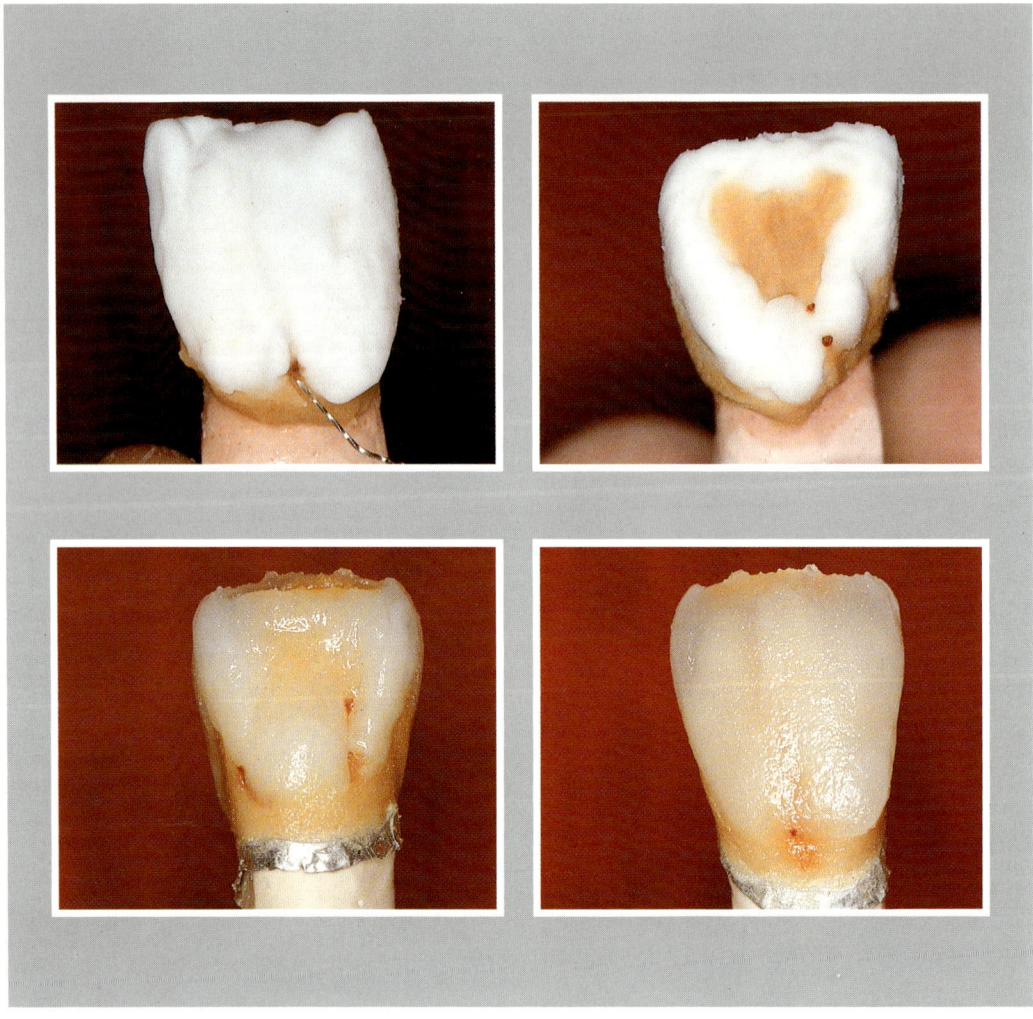

Figs 160 and 161   Occasionally brown spots or pits are required which may be built into the crown by an injection technique utilizing an endodontic reamer.

Figs 162 and 163   Here shown as a jacket crown After sintering all characteristics can be seen clearly.

Technique
After completion of the build-up an endodontic hand reamer No. 15 is used to inject Surface Stain of the correct colour into the crown (figs 160 to 163).

References

1. *Sozio R, and Sanderson A:* Quintessence of Dental Technology 10: 637, 1985.
2. *Yamamoto M:* Metal Ceramics. p 274. Chicago: Quintessence Publishing Co 1985.
3. *McLean J W:* The Future for Dental Porcelain p 33 to 34 in Dental Ceramics. ed. McLean J. W. Quintessence Publishing Co. 1983.
4. *Geller W:* Zurich. 2nd ISC Barbican. London 1984.

7 Occlusal Table of Posterior Teeth

Occlusal design is important for function and aesthetics. This chapter addresses the problems of accuracy in occlusion. The use of High Chroma Dentines is discribed to avoid opacity and provide aesthetic occlusal tables.

Building Technique for the Occlusal Table of Posterior Teeth Aesthetic Design

Even in the posterior region of the mouth aesthetic considerations are important. Teeth should not only function correctly but also appear natural. Often – due to insufficient space – an inadequate thickness of dentine and enamel results in occlusal tables appearing bright. Painting opaque modifiers in the fossae will help to overcome the high reflective nature of the opaque.

The use of High Chroma Dentines will give the illusion of depth with colour filtering through the fossae in a natural manner.

Occlusal staining, if required, should be subtle. Care to avoid staining every fissure of the anatomy will prevent the common appearance of a brown spider crawling across the occlusion.

Anatomy should resemble a tooth and be in harmony with the occlusal concept required for the patient.

In the case illustrated on the next five pages a cusp to fossae relationship is developed[1,2] with very light contact in group function on the working side and complete disclusion on the balancing side.

References

1. *Shillingburg H T, Hobo S, and Whitsett L D:* Fundamentals of Fixed Prosthodontics. p 235–245 Quintessence Publishing Co. 1978.
2. *Thomas P K:* Syllabus on Full Mouth Waxing Technique for Rehabilitation. San Diego Instant Printing Services. 1967.

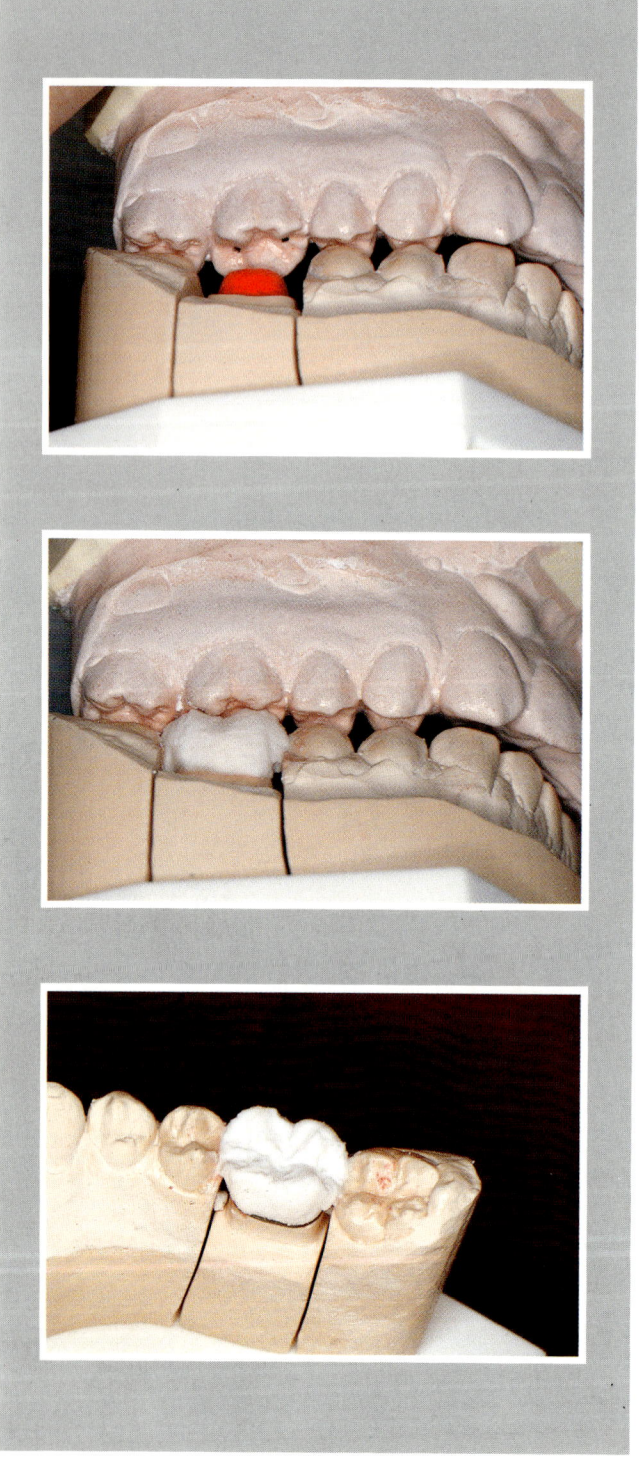

Fig 164   In this case a cusp to fossae relationship is indicated. To ensure that cusp tips are placed accurately into opposing fossae, a pencil mark is first placed to indicate the points of contact on the antagonist. Pencil is used at this stage so as not to prematurely discolour the porcelain. The incisal pin of the articulator is increased 1 mm to allow for shrinkage.

Fig 165   Dentine porcelain is added and the tooth anatomy is shaped. The buccal cusps are built into the position indicated by the pencil marks.

Fig 166   Occlusal anatomy is approximately shaped.

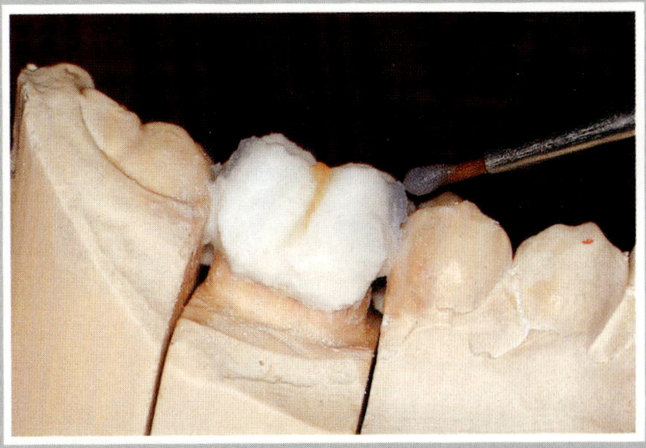

Fig 167 Facial techniques are similar to the anterior teeth. In this case CCS No. 7 Incisal Blue is placed mesially and distally at the cusp tips and CCS No. 16 Apricot is placed between the cusps. Color Clue Liquid is used to place these colours. Enamel overlays are used to complete the facial anatomy.

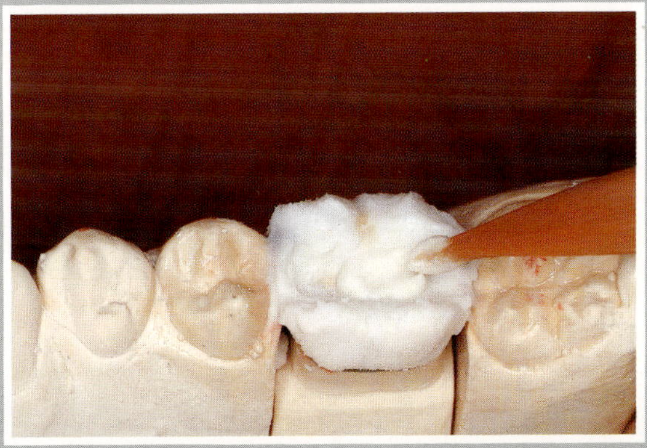

Fig 168 Occlusal depth of colour is achieved by cutting away dentine in the fossae and replacing with a High Chroma Dentine, in this case CCS 22 and Dentine 1:1.

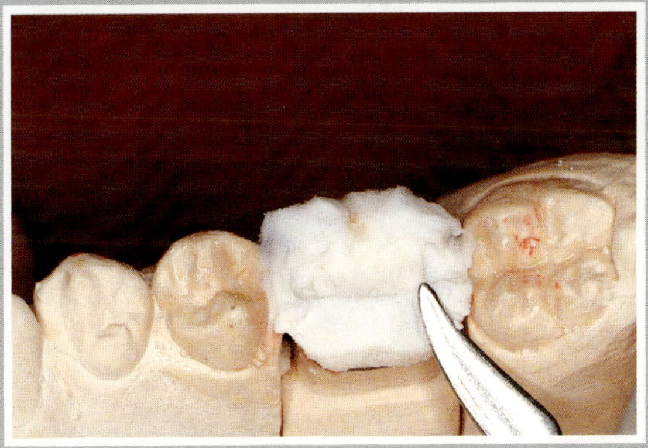

Fig 169 Lingual cusp tips are reduced to allow build-up in enamel porcelain.

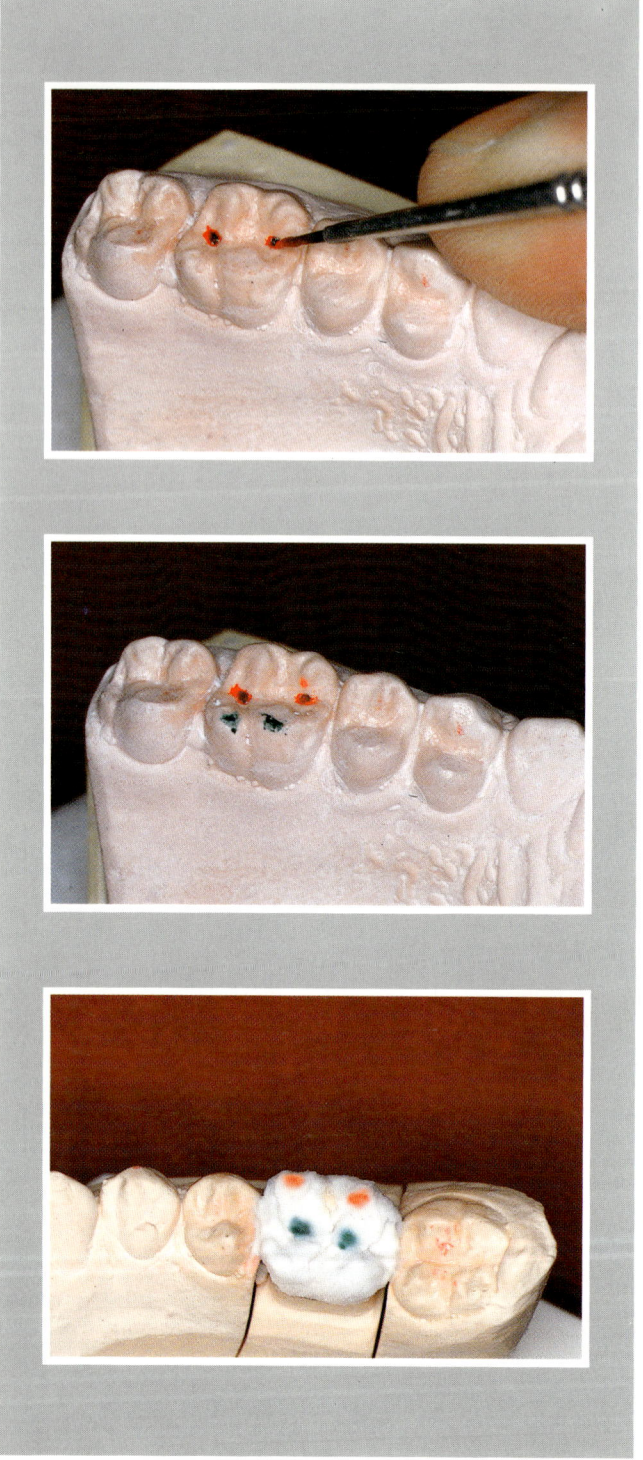

Fig 170 A small spot of red dye* is placed at each fossa in the same place as the pencil mark and cusp tips are built to contact.

Fig 171 The opposing mesial and distal palatal functioning cusp tips are marked with a green dye*.

Fig 172 Build-up is completed in S58 enamel porcelain. Red marks indicate buccal cusp contact with opposing maxillary fossae.
Green marks indicate contact of the maxillary palatal functioning cusps.

* Tanaka Bitex. Tanaka Dental Products. Skokie. Illionois 60077 USA

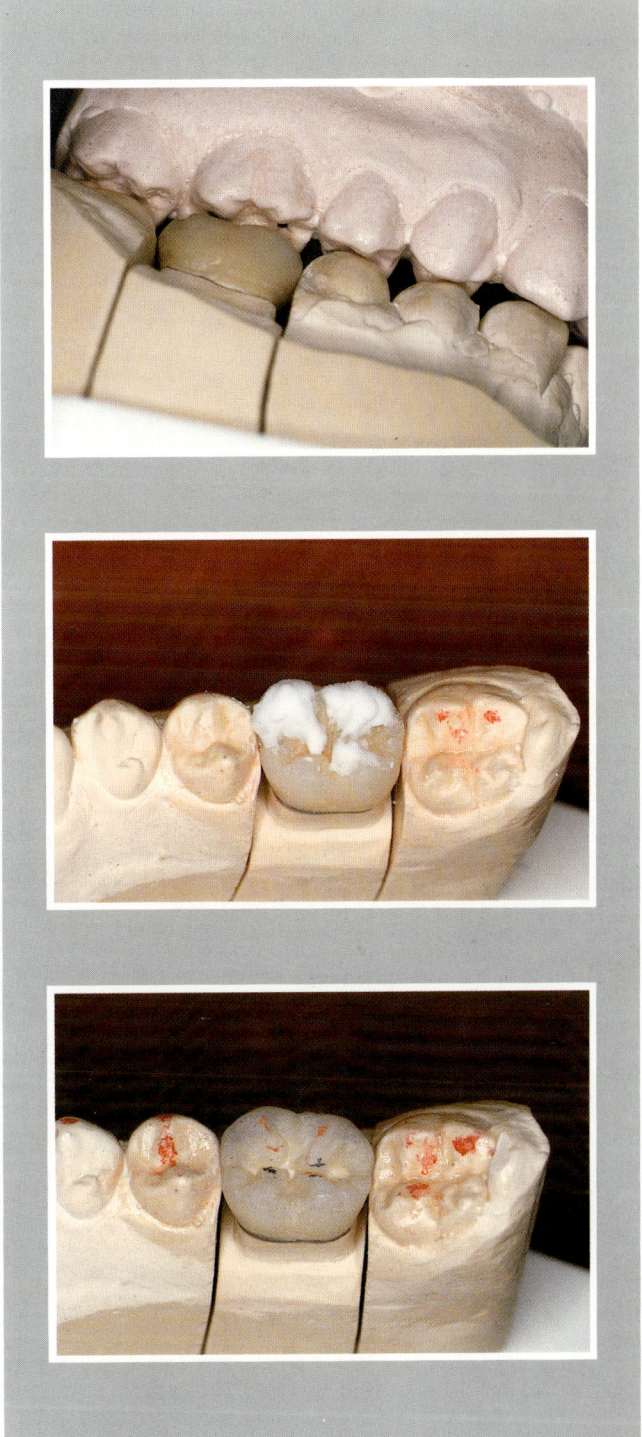

Fig 173 After sintering the incisal pin is reset and the crown is ground to fit. Cusp tips are correctly aligned but due to sintering contraction the mesial and distal buccal cusps are out of contact with the opposing fossae.

Fig 174 Additions are made in enamel porcelain. If an opalescent appearance is required transparent opalescent may be used at the cusp tips and ridges.

Fig 175 Occlusal adjustments are refined; only point contact is required with the opposing tooth. There is very light group function in working side excursion and no contact in balance excursion.

Note: Very often no contact in excursive movements is required in the posterior region, i.e. cuspid disclusion.

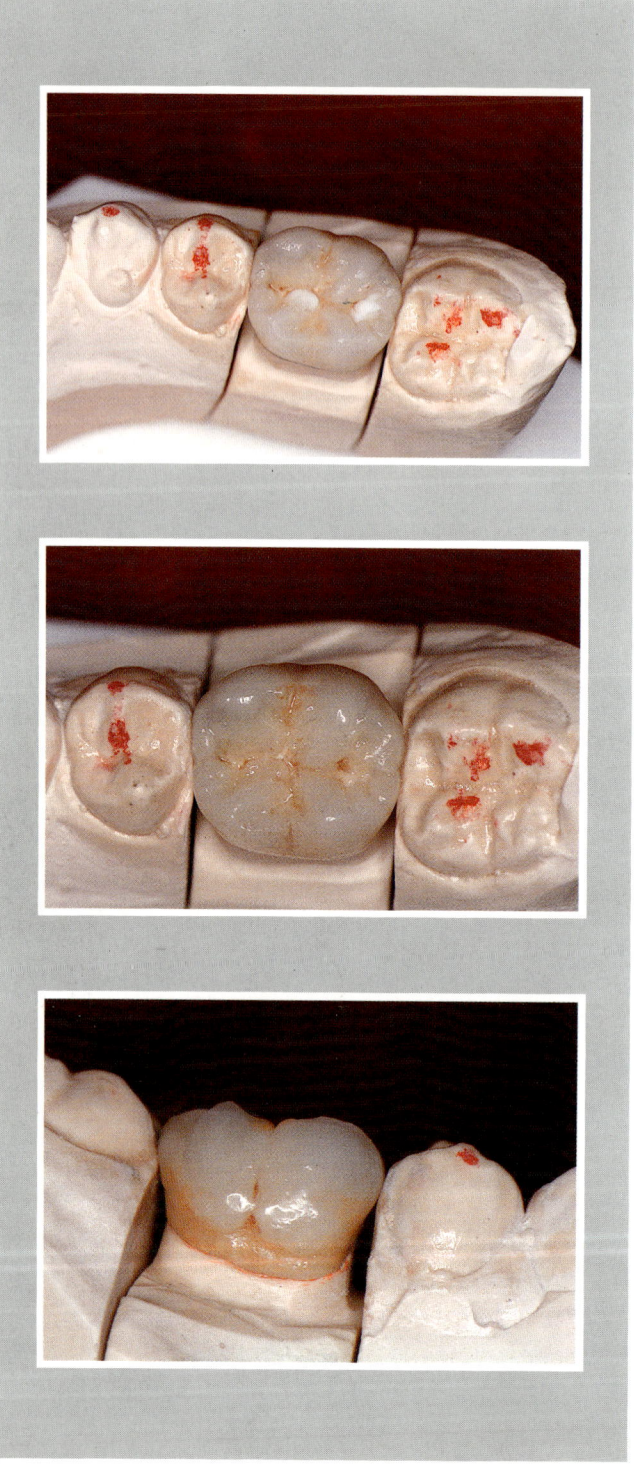

Fig 176 The crown is prepared for glazing. Surface stain is applied as necessary. Care should be taken to avoid over-emphasising the stain. An indication of the colour and degree of fissure stain given by the dentist will be a useful aid. Whilst stained teeth look attractive on the cast, they will look aesthetically poor in the mouth if out of character. Occasionally minor additions are necessary to close spaces between triangular ridges or to achieve fine contact with opposing dentition. These are added at this stage using enamel powder and Integral Corrector Opal 2:1.

Fig 177 Finished restoration. On the occlusal surface note the chroma filtering through the fissures giving depth and avoiding the need to use excessive surface stain.

Fig 178 Buccal view. Note: Blue cusp tip margins, opalescence in the cervical third and root formation, surface stain has been added between the cusps.

8 Posterior Tooth Form

Posterior tooth morphology is important to the maintenance of occlusion and periodontal health. Attention to such detail as occlusal contacts, tooth contact areas and axial wall profile help to maintain dental health in these vital areas.

The correct formation of tooth contours will in addition aid aesthetics as even in this region restorations should still look as natural as the tooth structure they are replacing.

8.1 Tooth Morphology

The importance of studying basic tooth shapes for the maintenance of the periodontium, the supporting muscles, and the temporomandibular joint (TMJ) in relation to the aesthetics involved is often overlooked during the fabrication of fixed prosthodontics.

The problem is that technicians do not study tooth morphology but rather rely on copying the teeth on the cast. Restorations must be in harmony with the rest of the dentition as well as the periodontium, the TMJ and the musculature. Often teeth copied on the cast have already had some form of restorative work – crowns and bridges, amalgam or composite fillings or just edentulous areas. In many cases the previous work is not anatomically correct or even biologically suitable. Therefore merely copying poorly shaped restorations leads to even poorer new restorations. By using this method technicians fail to learn correct tooth morphology, either because of the previous poor dentition or because detailed tooth anatomy is not very obvious on stone casts. These factors contribute to a poor understanding of tooth anatomy by many dental technicians.

One can draw an analogy with the knowledge and ability of a child whose understanding of human form is complete but basic. To use the human face as a yardstick our child could draw a reasonable line drawing (fig. 179). This simple sketch demonstrates good contour: the head is the correct shape, with accurate placement and alignment of ears, eyes, nose and mouth. Compare this with the poor sketch of the human face. This represents a similar accuracy to that of today's general standard. Poor contour and line angles have misshapen the outline of the head, there is inaccurate positioning of the facial features (ears, eyes etc.) and the left ear is missing. This may seem an extreme example but when compared to the diagrams in figs 180 and 181 it can be seen that many salient features are lacking: axial wall profile is often incorrect, occlusal anatomy inaccurate, triangular ridge, fissures and fossae either poorly shaped and at the wrong angle or entirely missing.

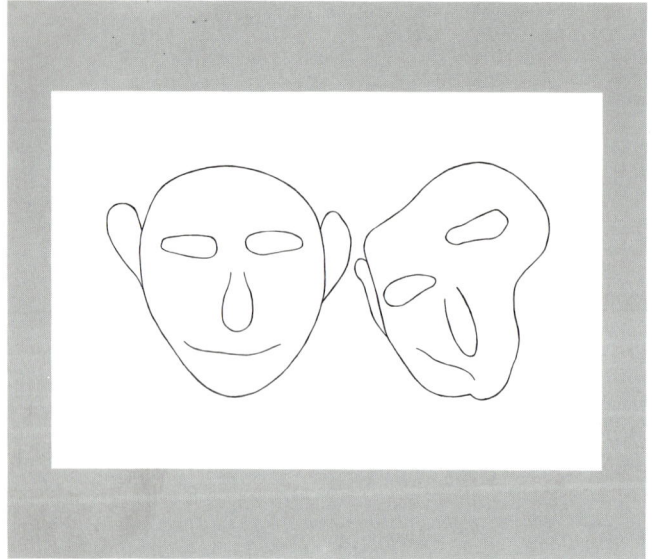

Fig 179 Left: Sketch of the human face, as drawn by a child. At an early age we can recognise and draw simple anatomy and familiar objects. We have the basic knowledge of facial contour and of position and angle of anatomical details such as ears, eyes, mouth etc.

Right: Misshapen sketch represents an analogy with dental restorations and the consequences of poor contour, misposition and incorrect angulation of basic features, common in many restorations.

Compare figs 180 and 181:

Fig 180 (left) Common mistakes in morphology result in a poor tooth shape, when compared with fig 181.

Fig 181 (right) Good contour, position and angulation of cusps and fissures.

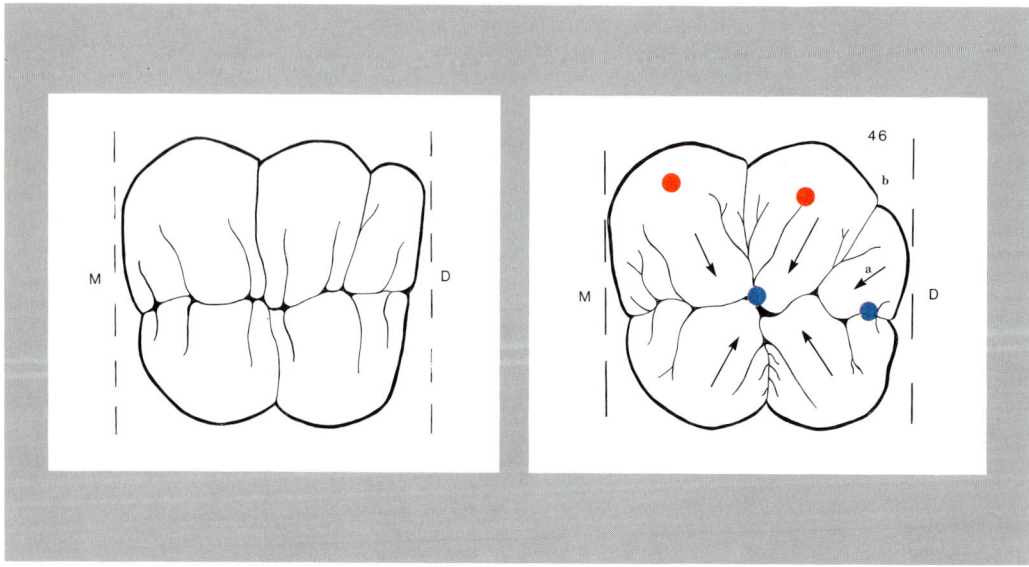

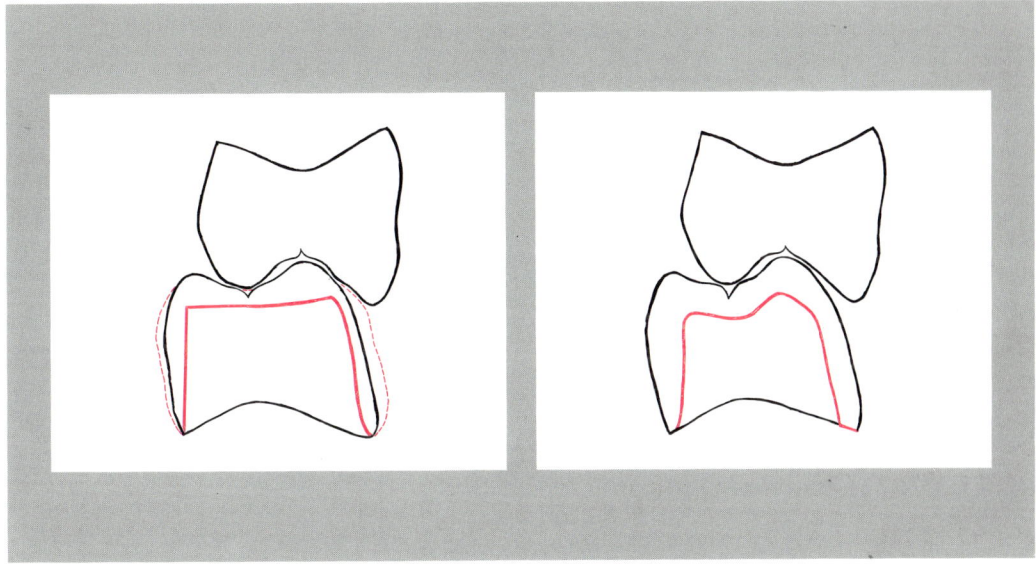

Fig 182 (left) Poor tooth reduction creates problems: either the ceramist compromises on the thickness of porcelain, resulting in an opaque appearance, or he over-contours. The only solution is to re-prepare allowing adequate room for metal/porcelain thickness of 1.3 mm – 1.5 mm.

Fig 183 (right) Preparation for ideal metal-ceramic thickness contours.

A team approach

The dental team approach to the problem can be divided into two areas: the clinical preparation, and the ability of the technician to understand basic tooth morphology.

Clinical preparation

The clinical preparation should ensure that there is adequate room for the technician to form correct axial wall profiles. Lack of attention to this aspect results in the following problems, which may in turn lead to periodontal involvement.
1. Grossly overcontoured axial walls
2. Wide occlusal tables
3. Poor aesthetics
4. Narrowing of the embrasure spaces
5. Accentuation of the suprabulge
 In addition, insufficient reduction in the areas of occlusal involvement may result in the following.
1. Increased tooth stress

2. TMJ problems
3. Poor aesthetics
4. Decreased masticatory ability
 In fixed prosthodontics correct tooth reduction should allow room for metal or porcelain or both in the case of a metal ceramic restoration. Figures 182 and 183 illustrate where judicious preparation allows room at the labio-occlusal line angle, the occlusal table, and at the preparation margin. It should be remembered that adequate clearance should be allowed in all eccentric mandibular movements.

 Dental technicians should study tooth morphology in order to improve aesthetics and to be aware of the effect that the restoration will make to the supporting tissues, periodontium, TMJ and musculature.

 The following factors are critical to the long-term success and acceptability of the restoration.

97

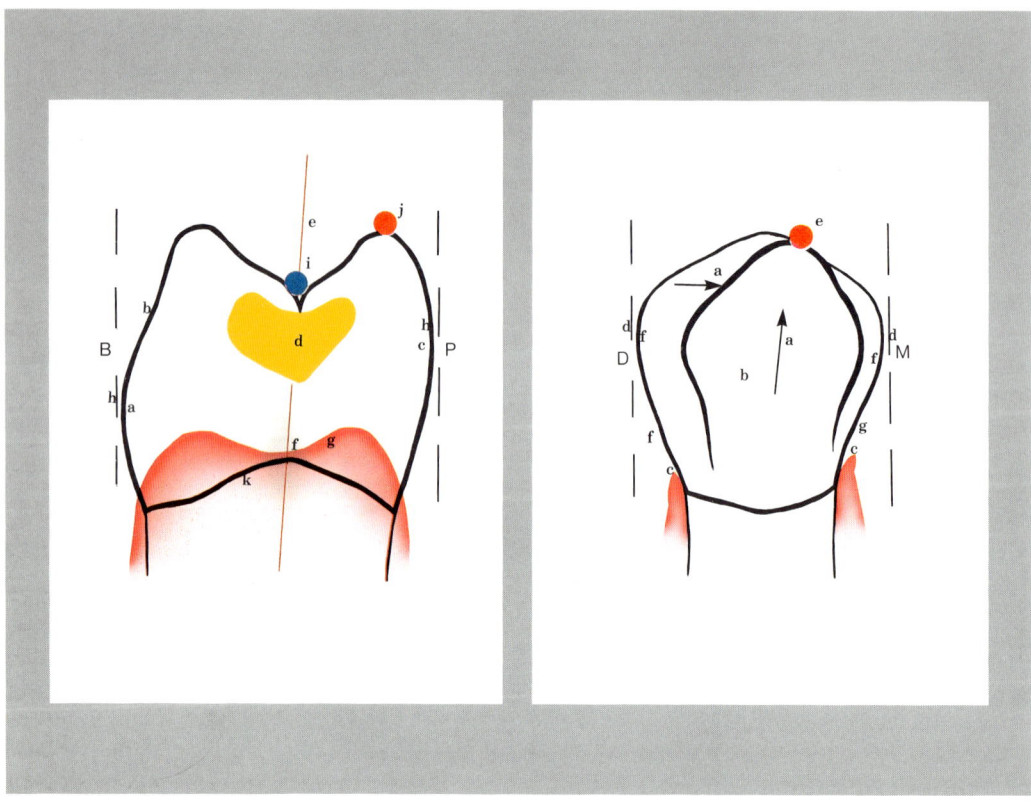

Atlas of Tooth Anatomy

In these examples most of the points to look for will be noted and therefore will not be repeated in subsequent examples.

Maxillary First Pre-molar

Figs 184 and 185

Fig 184   Left: Lateral Aspect.
a Buccal suprabulge
b Depression at the middle third
c Palatal contour is curved
d Contact area
e Tooth axis
f Proximal depression
g Tissue contour
h Height of contour
i Occluding area for mandibular cusp
j Occluding cusp
k Cementum enamel junction (CEJ)

Right: Palatal Aspect.
a Mesial positioning of palatal cusp (arrows)
b Small dimension of palatal cusp
c Free gingiva
d Height of contour
e Occluding cusp
f Convex contour
g Concave contour

1. Natural aesthetics
2. Tissue compatibility
3. Functional harmony

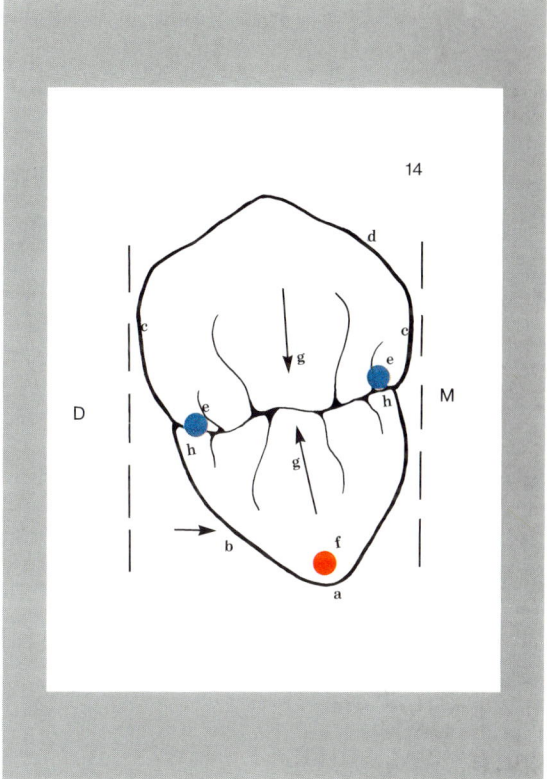

Fig 185 Occlusal Aspect.
a Mesial positioning of palatal cusp (arrow); compare with second pre-molar
b Mesial slope of palatal cusp marginal ridge
c Height of contour
d Contour line
e Occluding area of mandibular cusp (cusp to marginal ridge)
f Occluding cusp
g Cuspal angulation (arrows)
h Marginal ridge position
Note: Fissure pattern and cuspal angulation.

1. Natural aesthetics are important if the patient is to accept the restoration's appearance and be sufficiently confident to laugh and smile.

2. Axial wall line angles and embrasure spaces critical to the controlled displacement of the food bolus should prevent impaction between teeth or stagnation areas where debris can accumulate. The ability for the patient to clean between teeth and practise good oral hygiene is of paramount importance.

3. Recognised occlusal concepts must be adhered to, areas of occlusal contact and disclusion should be known as well as paths of movement. Occlusal tables of posterior teeth and the palatal inclines of upper anterior teeth must be designed with these concepts in mind.

8.2 Posterior tooth Details

Maxillary First Pre-Molar

Facial Profile
Facially the tooth resembles a canine. The cusp tip height of contour is placed distal to the tooth centre, the reverse cuspal angulation to the canine.

Developmental lobes and groves are evident.

Height of contour is in the middle third of the tooth.

Mesial and distal concavities are present at the cervical third.

Lateral Aspect
Palatal cusp tip is slightly shorter than the buccal cusp.

Buccal cusp is sharp as it is a shearing

cusp whilst the palatal cusp is rounded as it is the occluding cusp.

At the buccal face a suprabulge is evident coronal to the Cementum Enamel Junction (CEJ) with a depression at the middle third of the tooth face; the cervical incisal plane of the tooth face is flat. Height of contour is at the suprabulge. Palatally the tooth wall is slightly rounded with height of contour in the middle third.

Contact area is between the occlusal and body third of the tooth. Note the shape of the interdental papilla. A slight concavity is present at the cervical third approximating to the interdental papilla.

Buccal and palatal marginal ridges meet in a small notch (fig 184).

Palatal Aspect
The palatal cusp is shorter than the buccal and its long axis inclines mesially. The mesial bulge of the buccal cusp may be seen. The palatal cusp tip is mesially placed with a short steep slope towards the mesial and a long slope towards the distal. All contours

are rounded. This is in contrast to the palatal view of the buccal cusp tip which has the reverse contour (fig 184).

Occlusal Aspect
The occlusal is kidney-shaped, having a concave side mesially and a convex side placed distally. The wide buccal cusp is opposed by a smaller mesially inclined palatal cusp tip (fig 185).

Maxillary Second Pre-Molar

Basic tooth form is the same as the first premolar. The following differences should be noted.

Mesial distal width and bucco-palatal width is smaller. Palatal cusp is more centrally positioned with less of a mesial incline. Buccal and palatal cusps are of a more even size although the palatal cusp is still smaller.

Central fossa does not extend as far towards the marginal ridges (figs 186 and 187).

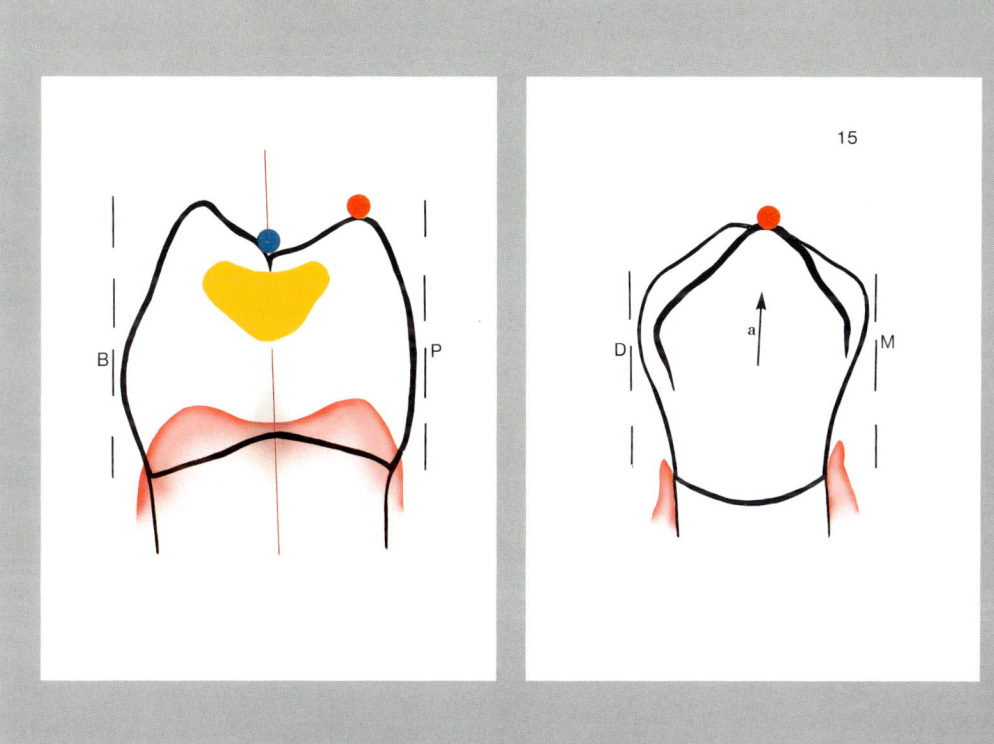

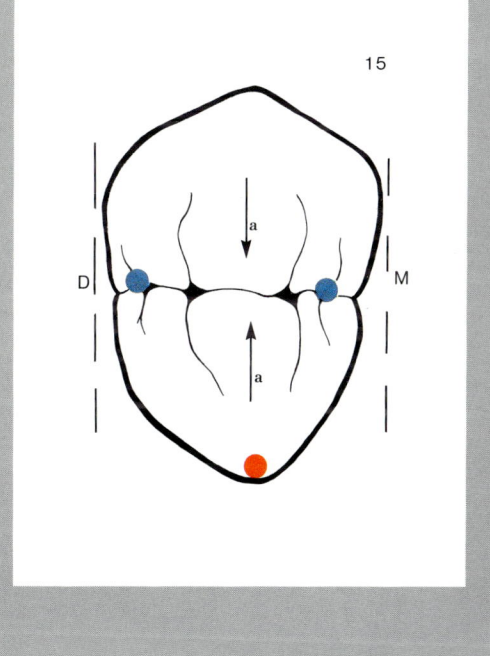

In the following examples further details pertinent to the individual tooth will be described.

Maxillary Second Pre-molar

Figs 186 and 187
Fig 186 Above Left: Lateral Aspect
Similar to first pre-molar.

Fig 186 Above Right: Palatal Aspect
a Angulation of palatal cusp is in line with tooth
   axis (arrow)
Note: large palatal cusp (compare with first pre-molar).

Fig 187 Occlusal Aspect:
Similar to first pre-molar with the exception of the palatal cusp which is aligned with the buccal cusp.
a (Arrows)

Maxillary First Molar

Facial Profile
– A double cusp facial aspect with a notched division.
– The mesial portion is larger and more dominant than the distal.
– A concavity exists at the mesial margin in the cervical region; a more rounded profile exists at the distal margin.
– Note the areas of greatest convexity.
– Tooth axis is angled mesially.

Lateral Aspect
Angulation of buccal and palatal walls allow proper displacement of food and good gingival stimulus, without food impaction into the gingival crevice.
– A suprabulge above the CEJ. is evident.
– Buccal cusps are more pointed and slightly longer than palatal cusps.
– Buccal cusps are the working cusps.
– Palatal cusps are the occluding cusps and therefore rounded.
– Buccal and palatal marginal ridges meet in a small notch.
– Buccal wall profile is straight with only a slight deviation towards the palatal aspect.
– A depression exists at the middle of the buccal wall.
– Palatal wall profile is rounded.
Distal wall is smaller and more rounded than the mesial.
– Contact area is between the occlusal and body third of the tooth (fig. 188).

Palatal Aspect
– The mesial cusp is markedly larger than the distal and has a mesial inclination.
– Mesial cusp often carries an accessory cusp termed the cusp of Carabelli.
– Palatal width is less than the buccal facial width.
– The tooth tapers towards the cervix.
– A mesial concavity and distal convexity are evident (fig 188).

Occlusal Aspect
The occlusal table is divided into two distinct sections. The trigon includes the mesio-buccal, disto-buccal and mesio-palatal cusps. The talon bears the remaining disto-palatal cusp. The junction between the trigone and the talon is marked by a distinct groove almost bisecting the tooth, passing at an oblique angle from the mesio-palatal cusp to the disto-buccal cusp.
– Occlusal outline is rhomboidal in shape with the buccal width obviously wider than the palatal profile.
– The mesial and distal marginal ridges angle in a disto-palatal direction.
– Mesial tooth width is greater than distal tooth width.
– The tooth appears to angle towards the mesio-buccal cusp.
– The mesio-palatal cusp dominates the occlusal table whilst the disto-palatal cusp is the most inferior of the four cusps.
– Mesial marginal ridge is concave and the distal marginal ridge is convex.
– Buccal and palatal marginal ridges meet in a small notch.
– Occasionally secondary tubercles may be present at the mesial marginal ridge. These are not evident at the distal marginal ridge[1] (fig 189).

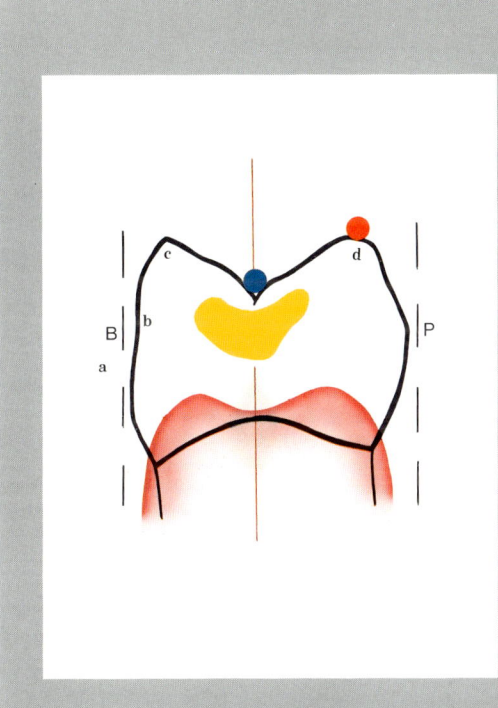

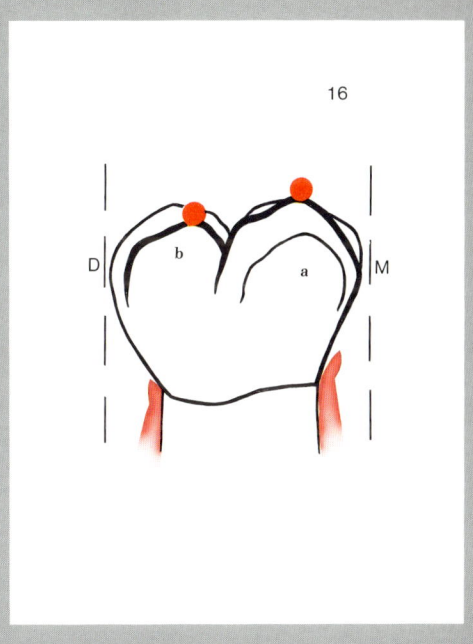

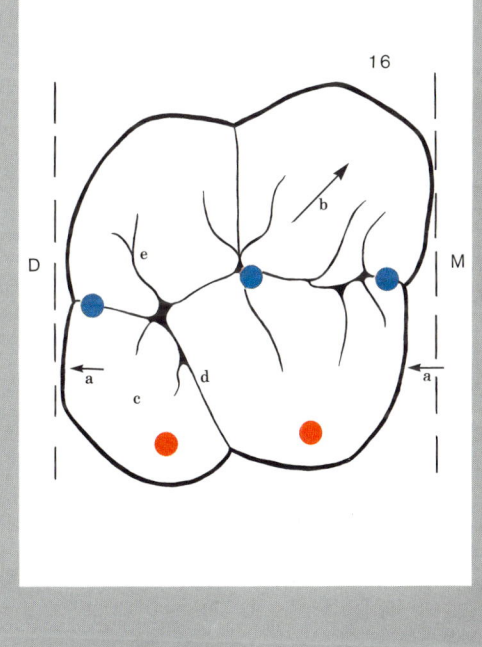

Maxillary First Molar

Figs 188 and 189
Fig 188   Above Left: Lateral Aspect
a   Buccal wall angulation is almost vertical
b   Depression above the suprabulge
c   Cusp tip is pointed due to shearing action
d   Palatal cusp tip is rounded due to occlusal wear
Applies to all maxillary posterior teeth.

Fig 188   Above Right: Palatal Aspect
a   Cusp of Carabelli
b   Disto-palatal cusp (compare size with second
    molar)

Fig 189   Occlusal Aspect
a   Mesial and distal margins angle towards the
    palate in a distal direction (arrows)
b   Mesio-buccal angulation of whole occlusal sur-
    face.
c   Compare size of disto-palatal cusp with second
    molar.
d   Transverse groove
e   Disto-buccal cusp accessory fissure continues
    from transverse groove

Maxillary Second Molar

Basic form is the same as the first molar. The following differences should be noted.

The tooth dimensions are smaller. Viewed from the occlusal, the distal wall and marginal ridge are convex with a distinct rounding towards the mesial at the disto-palatal corner. As a result the disto-palatal cusp is much smaller. No cusp of Carabelli exists (figs 190 and 191).

Maxillary Third Molar

This tooth has a variety of forms. Although it often resembles the second molar, the profile is coronet shaped with a deep central fissure.

In restorative practice the form of the second molar is a useful gide.

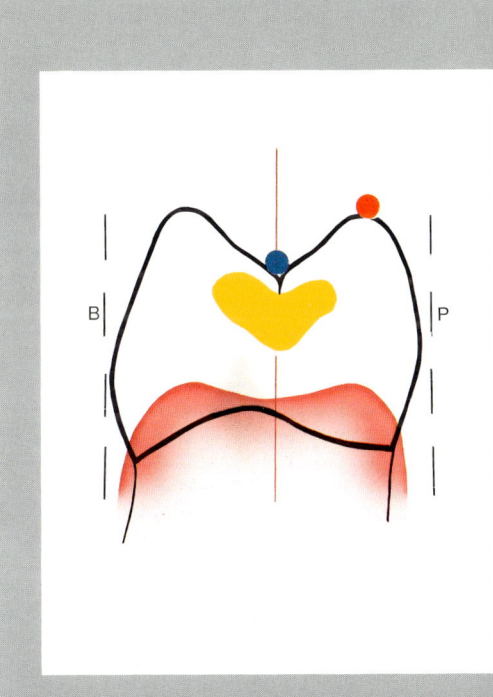

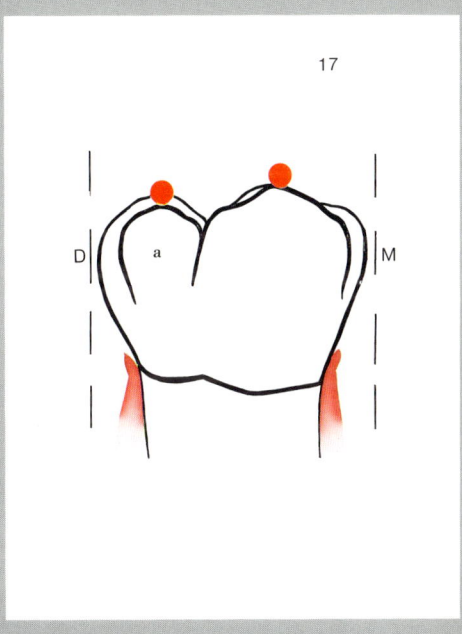

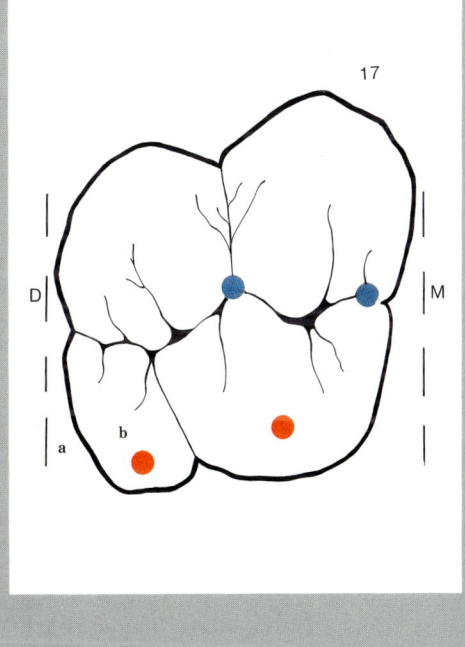

Maxillary Second Molar

Figs 190 and 191
Fig 190 Above Left: Lateral Aspect
Similar to maxillary first molar, no cusp of Carabelli
is present.

Fig 190 Above Right: Palatal Aspect
a Small disto-palatal cusp

Fig 191 Occlusal Aspect
a Mesial curve of distal margin (compare with first
molar)
b Small disto-palatal cusp (compare with first molar)

Mandibular First Pre-Molar

Facial Profile
- Triangular-shaped, similar to mandibular canine but with a flatter cusp tip contour, which is often rounded through abrasion as this is the occluding cusp.
- Height of tip contour is towards the mesial with a longer slope towards the distal.
- The mesial side is convex with only a slight concavity at the cervical third, whilst the distal side is convex with a slightly larger concavity at the cervical third.
- Height of contour of the facial aspect is in the cervical third.
- The developmental lobe and grooves are evident at the occlusal third.

Lateral Aspect
- The inferior lingual cusp may be seen clearly.
- Buccal cusp occupies two thirds of bucco-lingual width.
- The lingual inclination of this tooth can be seen.

- Height of contour on the facial aspect is in the cervical third.
- The lingual wall contour is flat and generally vertical in its sagittal plane.

This tooth differs from all other posterior teeth due to the lack of an occlusal table. The lingual cusp is markedly small and is marked by a groove which transverses the mesial marginal ridge.
- The buccal cusp tip is rounded as it is the occluding cusp.
- The buccal cusp takes up approximately two-thirds of the bucco-lingual width.
- Contact areas are located in the occlusal third (fig 192).

Lingual Occlusal Aspect
The inferior lingual cusp is evident allowing the larger buccal cusp to be seen from this aspect. A triangular ridge extends from the buccal cusp tip to the small lingual cusp.
- Fossae are present either side.
- The distal side is larger than the mesial (Fig 193).

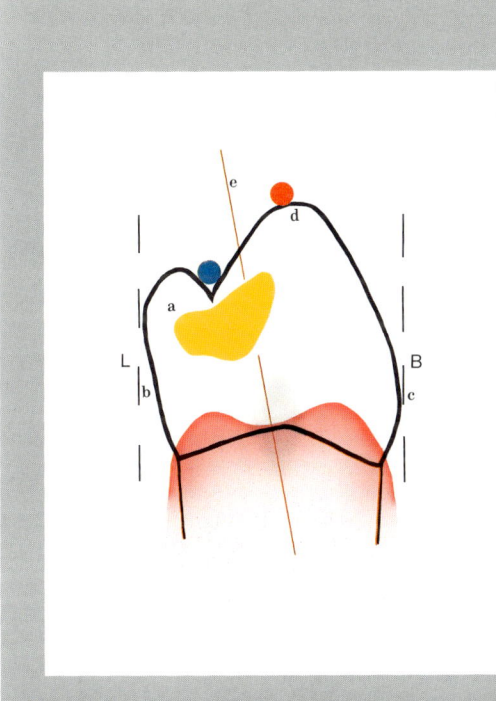

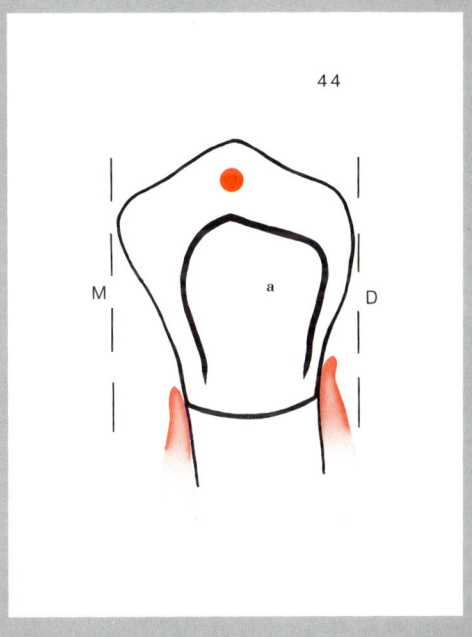

Mandibular First Pre-molar

Figs 192 and 193
Fig 192 Above Left: Lateral view
a Very small and low lingual cusp
b Flat lingual wall profile
c Buccal wall height of contour at cervical third
d Rounded buccal cusp tip due to occlusal wear
e Lingual angulation of tooth

Above Right: Lingual Aspect
a Small dimension of lingual cusp

Fig 193 Occlusal Aspect
a Small dimension of lingual cusp
b Mesial margin tapers (arrow)
c Central fissure often traverses the mesial marginal ridge creating a small depression

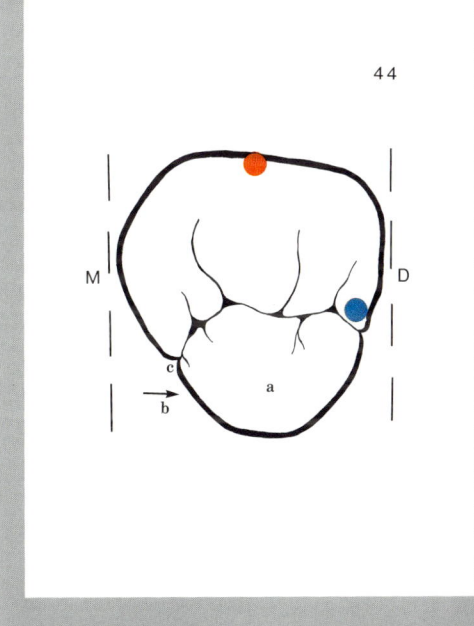

Mandibular Second Pre-Molar

Facial Profile
Compared to the first pre-molar the facial aspect is a little shorter but otherwise it is the same.

Lateral Aspect
Buccal cusp tip is higher than the lingual. Height of contour of the buccal wall is in the cervical region and the lingual angulation is evident.

Lingual wall is flat or with slight convex contour. Height of contour is in the middle third.

Buccal cusp tip is slightly higher than the lingual and is rounded as this is the occluding cusp.

Lingual cusps are large compared to the first pre-molar. The bucco-lingual width is greater than the first pre-molar and appears rectangular.

Buccal cusp occupies approximately three-fifths of the occlusal width (fig 194).

Lingual Aspect
Lingual morphology varies considerably. The lingual wall may be divided creating two separate cusps but often the separation is ill-defined and appears as a depression. Occasionally a single cusp exists.

Where two cusps exist it is the mesial which is the larger with the divide occurring distal to the centre. The tooth tapers towards the cervix (fig 194).

Occlusal Aspect
Where the morphology includes a lingual double cusp the occlusal outline is square. Single lingual cusp morphology presents a rounded outline. Double cusps may be observed with a more dominant mesial cusp.

Buccal and lingual marginal ridges are almost parallel with a slight taper to the lingual and meet in a notch. Note cuspal anatomy and position and direction of fissure and fossae (fig 195).

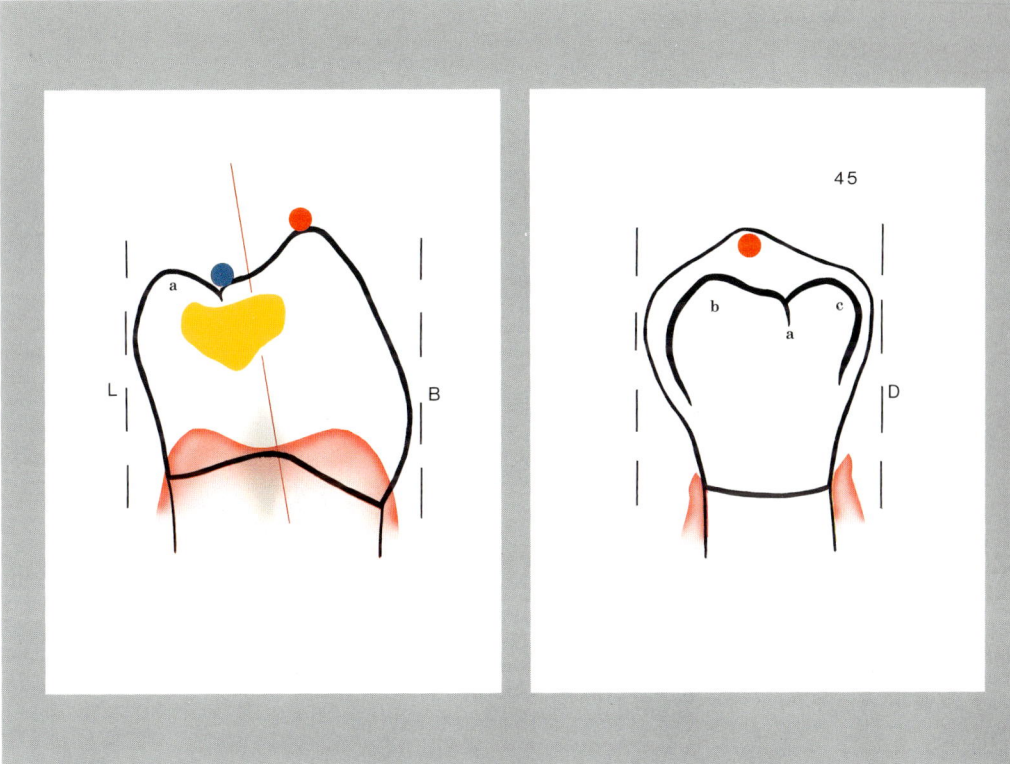

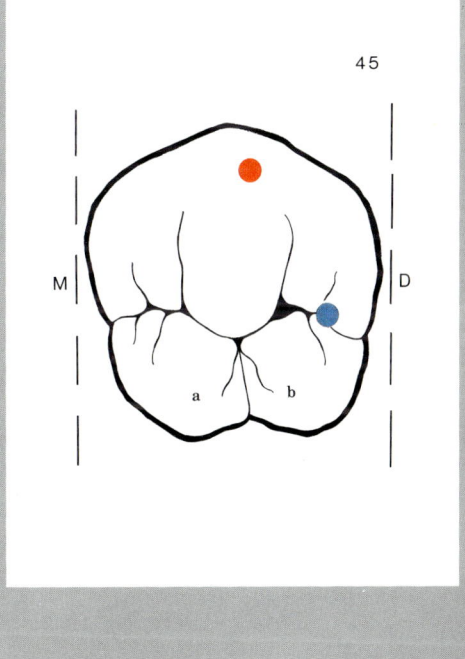

Mandibular Second Pre-molar

Figs 194 and 195
Fig 194 Above Left: Lateral Aspect
Buccal cusp is larger than lingual
a Lingual cusp height is at occlusal plane

Fig 194 Above Right: Lingual Aspect
a Lingual cusp is occasionally divided by a depression placed towards the distal aspect
b The mesio-lingual cusp is larger than the disto-lingual cusp (c).

Fig 195 Occlusal Aspect
Note square profile
a Mesio-lingual cusp
b Disto-lingual cusp

Mandibular First Molar

Facial Profile
Three cusp contours are present. The dominant cusp may be either the mesio-buccal or the disto-buccal cusp. The third cusp is placed at the disto-buccal corner and is inferior to the two major buccal cusps in size and height. A larger mesial wall concavity exists at the cervical third compared to the distal wall profile. The tooth is wider at the cervix than maxillary molars, thereby giving the tooth a rectangular appearance.

Note the height of contour at the mesial and distal margins. Cusp tips are flattened by wear as these are the occluding cusps.

The CEJ is peaked in an apical direction between the cusps.

Lateral Aspect
The entire tooth angles towards the lingual aspect in harmony with the curve of Monson and to interdigitate with opposing maxillary teeth.

A buccal suprabulge is evident occlusal to the CEJ

Buccal height of contour is at the cervical third and in the occlusal third on the lingual aspect.

Buccal cusps are flattened by wear, being the occluding cusps.

Lingual cusps are lower than buccal cusps and often more pointed due to their lingual non-working position to the maxillary palatal cusp.

Buccal and lingual marginal ridges meet in a small notch; the mesial notch is more pronounced.

Lingual profile is flat.

A concavity is present in the cervical third. Contact area is positioned between the occlusal and middle thirds (fig 196).

Lingual Aspect
Smaller than the buccal profile, two cuspal contours are evident. The cusp tips are more pointed than the buccal cusps.

The tooth has a wider cervix than the maxillary molar. The mesial cusp is slightly longer than the distal (fig 196).

Occlusal Aspect
Buccal cusps dominate the lingual cusps in width and extend a little further than halfway across the occlusal table before meeting the lingual cusp in a central fossa. Note the angulation of the disto-buccal accessory cusp which often appears as an enlarged marginal ridge.

To accommodate this cusp the mesial to distal central fissure is angled lingually.

Bucco-lingual marginal ridges meet in a notch. The mesial notch is usually more pronounced.

The mesial marginal ridge is concave and the distal marginal ridge is convex.

Lingual triangular ridge angles are dependent upon inter-condylar width.

In most cases the mesio-lingual cusp is joined to the disto-buccal cusp across the central fossa (fig 197).

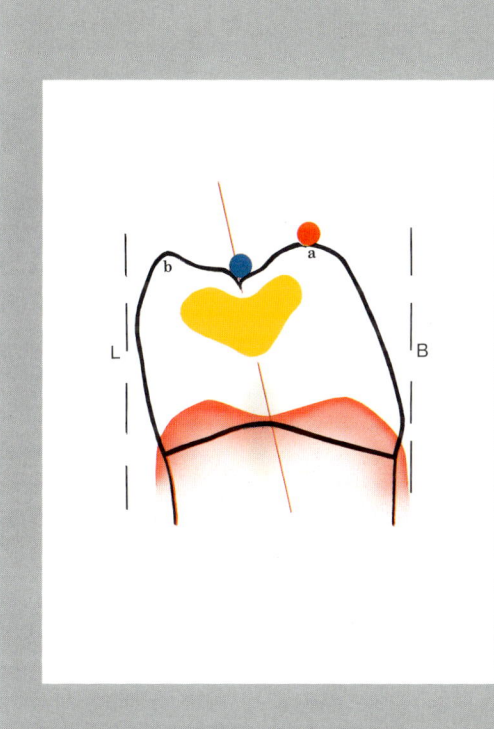

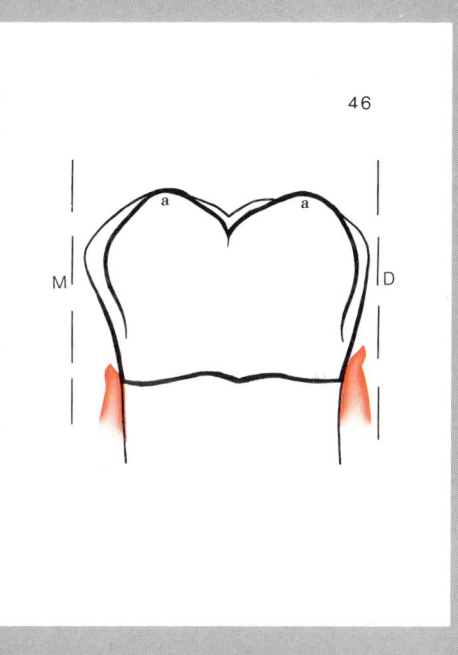

Mandibular First Molar

Figs 196 and 197
Fig 196 Above Left: Lateral Aspect
a Buccal cusps rounded due to occlusal wear
b Lingual cusps are pointed as they are not in occlusion

Fig 196 Above Right: Lingual Aspect
a Lingual cusps are pointed

Fig 197 Occlusal Aspect
a Note: the angulation of disto-buccal accessory cusp
b Round shape at disto-buccal margin
Note: angulation of cusps disto-buccal to mesio-lingual are in line whilst mesio-buccal and disto-lingual are not.

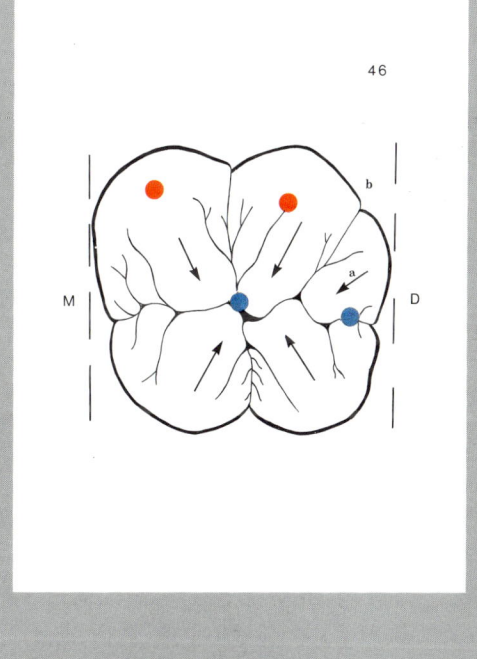

Mandibular Second Molar

Facial Profile
Similar to the first molar but smaller without the accessory disto-buccal cusp, so that the tooth is almost rectangular in outline.

Mesial and distal margin concavities in the cervical region are less than in other teeth creating a more ovoid facial appearance.

The CEJ is peaked apically between the cusps.

Lateral Aspect
Smaller than the first molar, otherwise similar in all other respects (fig 198).

Lingual Aspect
Similar to the first molar but due to the square shape of the tooth and the relative width of the facial aspect the buccal walls are not seen from this aspect.

Crown height is shorter than the first molar (fig 198).

Occlusal Aspect
This tooth is smaller than the first molar and the occlusal outline is almost square.

The fissure pattern is markedly different from the first molar, having no ancillary cusp at the distal aspect and a different cuspal arrangement.

Cusp anatomy is uniform with a cross shaped fissure pattern (fig 199).

Mandibular Third Molar

The tooth has a variety of forms although its general shape is that of the second molar.

Occlusal anatomy often exhibits four of five cusps with a deep central fissure.

In restorative practice the form of the second molar is a useful guide.

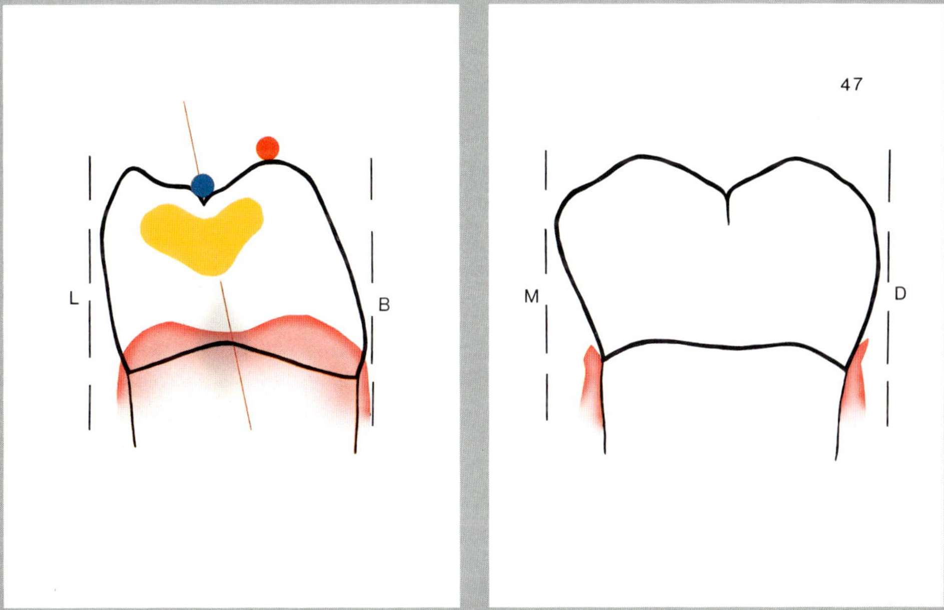

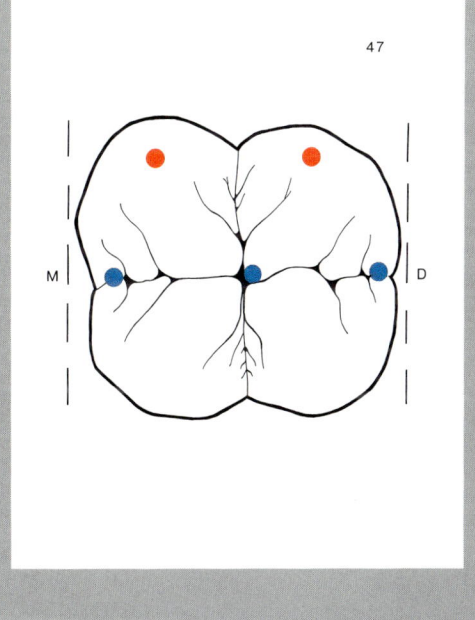

47

47

Mandibular Second Molar

Figs 198 and 199
Fig 198 Left and Right: Lateral and Lingual view
Compare contour with first molar.

Fig 199 Occlusal Aspect.
Compare contour with first molar.

References

1. *Berkovitz, Holland and Moxham:* Oral Anatomy. Wolfe Medical Publications Ltd.

Further Reading

Gründler H: The Study of Tooth Shapes. Quintessence Publishing Co. 1976.

Kuwata M: Color Atlas of Ceramo-Metal Technology. Vol 1. Ishiyaku Euro America, Inc. 1986.

Pokorny D K, and Blake F P: Principles of Occlusion. University of Detroit. Distributed by Denar Corporation. 1980

Renner R P: An Introduction to Dental Anatomy and Esthetics. Quintessence Publishing Co. 1985.

9 Finishing Techniques

Surface texture and lustre are important factors in the quality of the restoration. This chapter deals with the simulation of natural tooth surfaces.

9.1 Surface Definition

To attain natural character green abrasives, diamond points and wheels are used. A small diamond point is used to create a fine surface perikymata in harmony with the existing dentition, followed by an impregnated rubber wheel to smooth areas such as the heights of contour of the development lobes, marginal ridges and areas of abrasion (figs 200 to 203).

The selection of grinding instruments is important as differing particle size and wearing pattern of the abrasive will affect the surface finish. Rough diamonds and stones may cause the porcelain to chip and fine grains may detach from the surface leaving a roughened surface and small pits difficult to detect until after the glaze cycle.

In instances where the surface porcelain has been contaminated, either by silicone or rubber wheels which create a high surface tension, or by the restoration having been inserted into the mouth, then a light blasting with 25 μ aluminium oxide at 40psi is recommended to decontaminate the surface, followed by steam or ultrasonic cleaning (fig 204).

9.2 Surface Lustre

Ceramic surfaces which are highly glazed create high (specular) reflection which will mirror back light waves to the observer's eye, creating many problems. Natural dentition does not have the appearance of glass or of highly glazed porcelain, which often appears unnatural in the mouth. Surfaces therefore should be matched to natural conditions. When high surface reflection exists more light will be reflected back to the observer's eye causing a loss in depth of chroma and general translucency. Conversely if more light is allowed to penetrate deeper into the dentine layer then wherever the light waves penetrate the colour will be picked up and through diffused reflection transmitted back to the observer's eye.[1,2,3]

Where there is no light there can be no transmitted colour. By having a high reflective surface less light enters into the enamel and dentine layers beneath the surface thereby reducing depth of chroma. Surface polishing reduces surface reflection and natural tooth surfaces can be simulated (fig 205).

Smooth and polished enamel surfaces are common in the aged dentition. Attempting to simulate this by overglazing will result in a devalued colour tone and a highly reflective surface which will appear glass-like and

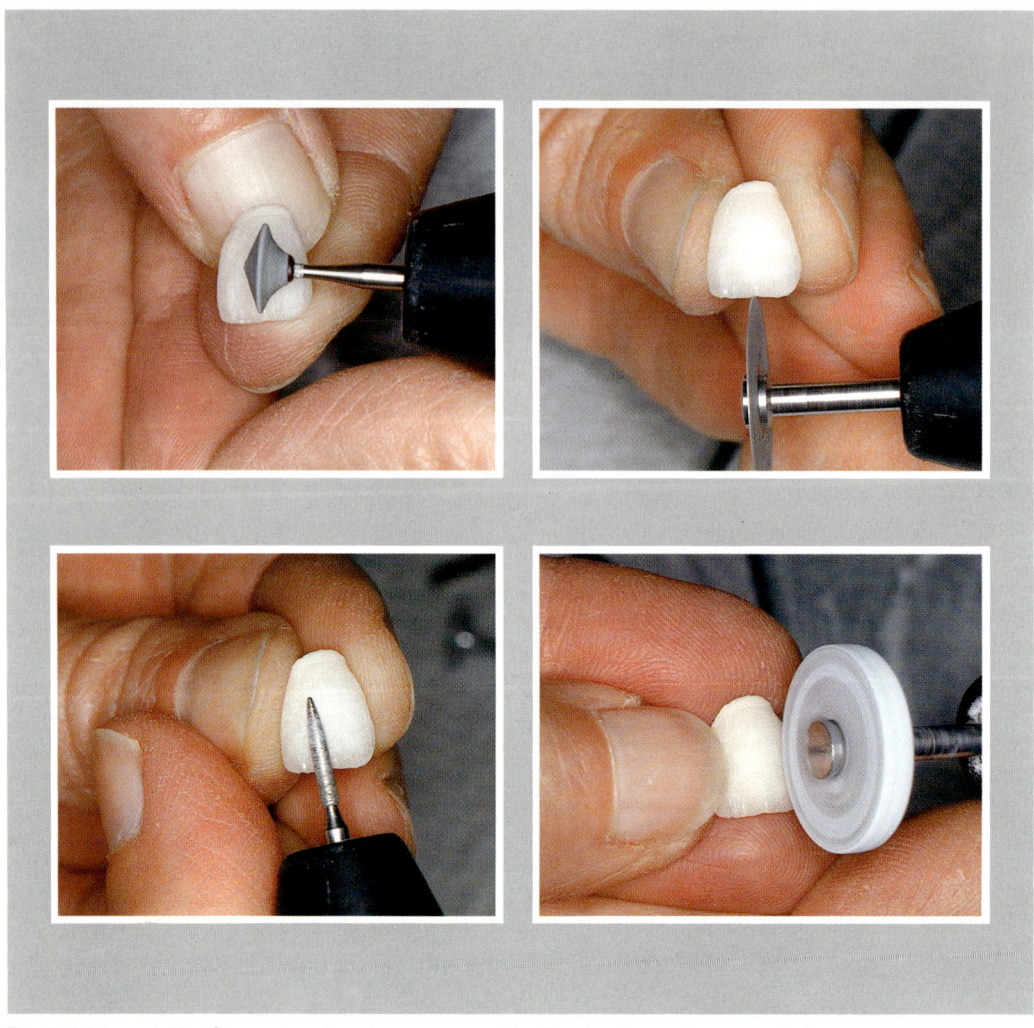

Fig 200 (above left)   Green abrasive stones are used to develop the surface morphology.

Fig 201 (above right)   Fine grooves and chipping at the incisal edge are made with a thin single sided diamond disc.

Fig 202 (below left)   Surface stria (perikymata) is produced with a medium grit diamond point.

Fig 203 (below right)   Height of contour, marginal areas and wear facets are smoothed with an impregnated rubber.*

---

* Exa Intrpol Polisher. Edenta AG Ch-9434 AN/SG Hauptstraße 7, St Gallen, Switzerland.

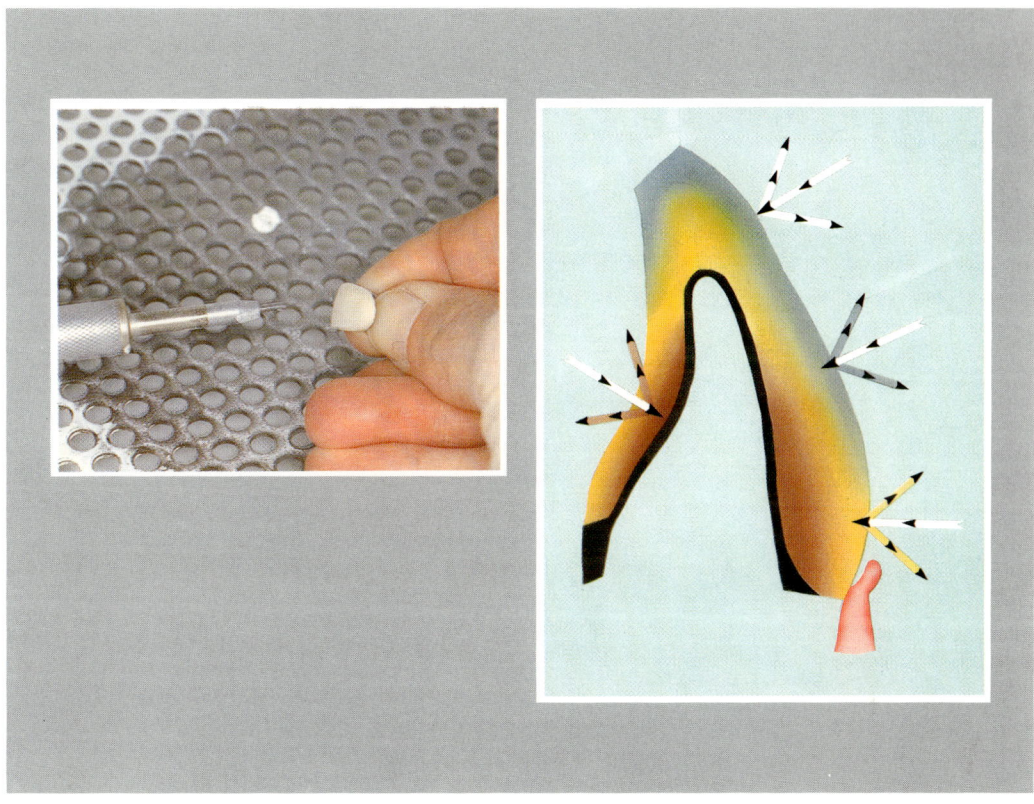

Fig 204 (left)   After using a rubber wheel it will be necessary to blast the surface with 25 μ aluminium oxide powder as the porcelain will have a high surface tension and the application of surface stains will be hindered.

Fig 205 (right)   Colour is perceived by its transmission back to the observer through diffused reflected light. In high glazed porcelain, surface reflection reduces the percentage of light passing through the surface. White arrow shows white light reflection from the surface.
Other arrows depict the way in which light enters the structure and colour is then reflected back.

unnatural in the mouth. A correctly glazed enamel will melt only to a depth of approximately 25 μ.[1]

Overglazed porcelain results in an amorphous glass which has lost the prismatic effect created by light reflection from the grain boundaries.[4]

It has been suggested that a low glaze resulting in a satin surface, followed by physical polishing of the ceramic to the desired degree of lustre, retains the prismatic quality of the grain boundary, and is the way to achieve the desired result.

With this technique a danger exists of over-polishing fine surface detail (perikymata). Difficulties in polishing interdental areas and occlusal contours could also present problems in maintaining oral hygiene.

Glaze – Polish Procedure

Normal glaze procedures followed by lightly polishing off the reflective glare of the glaze gives the desired results and maintains a surface glaze in all the areas where access is difficult for polishing.

Small alteration to colour of surface

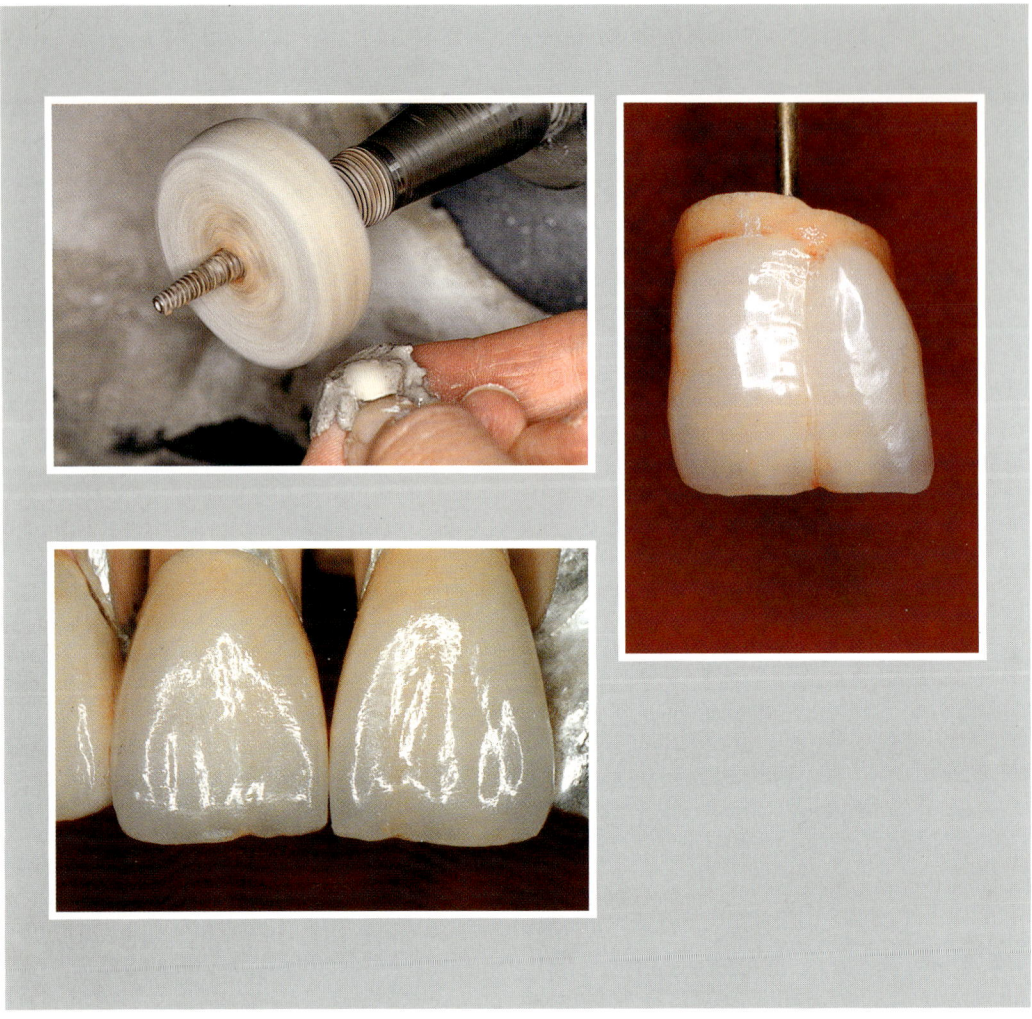

Fig 206 (above left)   A medium grit pumice is used with a felt wheel to remove the reflective glaze.

Fig 207 (below left)   Working case seen here on the cast demonstrates surface texture after glaze firing and prior to polishing with pumice. Note also the surface contour, developed by using the green abrasive as in *fig 200*.

Fig 208 (right)   Phantom case demonstrates natural surface after polishing with pumice.

characterising may be accomplished at this stage, bearing in mind that facial staining is contra-indicated as this will be polished after glaze and any surface stain will be removed.

Glazing procedures should allow the surface porcelain to exhibit a medium gloss, without loss of surface definition or rounding of line angles. High glazing is not recommended.

Polishing Technique

The action of polishing the ceramic surface with a felt wheel will smooth the many minute facets and grinding marks which may not be seen easily with the eye, but which leave the restoration appearing clumsy.

To assess the quality of surface texture a silicone impression of a completed restoration may be taken. Inspection of the resultant cast will serve as a useful guide to correct contour and also texture.

Using a polishing lathe and a 5 cm diameter felt wheel a technique similar to denture polishing is employed (fig 206), in which pumice is applied to the porcelain surface and the restoration is moved continuously in order to avoid creating lines.

By utilizing various polishing mediums it is possible to impart varying degrees of lustre.

A medium grit pumice imparts a satin finish evident in a high percentage of young to middle-aged dentitions (figs 207 and 208). Mixing the pumice with liquid metal polish[+] will create a high lustre. Diamond polishing paste applied with a 2.5 cm diameter felt wheel mounted on the handpiece increases the lustre still further, simulating the polished surfaces common in the elderly.

On no account should diamond paste be applied to a glazed surface as this will exaggerate the reflectivity. Surfaces should always be pumice polished first and, if required, further procedures should follow to increase lustre.

[+] Brasso. Reckitt Household Producs, Hill, England.

9.3 The Double Glaze Technique

It is not always possible to achieve total accuracy of colour without the use of surface stains, as basic hue may need slight alterations (only effective up to half shade). Subtle variation in zonal colouration and enhancement of inbuilt colours are often better effected with the double glaze technique.

As surface texture and lustre are important qualities a procedure is adopted which allows both the glaze and polish techniques and surface staining.

After checking contour the surface is prepared taking care to create a similar stria pattern (perikamata) to the rest of the dentition.

Some surface staining may be carried out at the first glaze stage. Areas that will be unaffected by the polishing technique such as embrasures, occlusal and lingual aspects may be enhanced with stain at this stage.

Glazing is carried out followed by polishing of the ceramic surface until the desired degree of lustre is achieved.

Surface stains are now applied as necessary and a low second glaze is achieved at 850 °C, which will raise the surface lustre slightly.

A restoration with harmonious surface texture and lustre will result whilst maintaining optimal shade control.

References

1. *McLean J W:* Science and Art Vol 1. p 122–125. Quintessence Publishing Co. 1979.
2. *Preston J D:* Color and Esthetics in Dental Porcelain p 308. The State of the Art 1977. Ed. Yamada H. N. University of Southern California.
3. *Clarke F J J:* Measurement of Color of Human Teeth p 449–455 in Dental Ceramics Proceedings of the First International Symposium on Ceramics. Ed. McLean J. W. Quintessence Publishing Co. 1983.
4. *McLean J W:* Science and Art Vol II. p 25. Quintessence Publishing Co. 1980.

10 Phantom Cases

The following phantom cases are illustrated to show the many characteristic details and aesthetic possibilities.

10.1 Characteristic Details for Maxillary Anterior Porcelain Jacket Crowns

Young Dentition

Each tooth is built to simulate different conditions and the canine has been built one shade darker.

Maxillary central displays the typical mamelon arrangement together with a translucent incisal with blue extending down the marginal ridges and a dentine coloured halo effect.

Maxillary lateral is similar to the central but has only two mamelons. White enamel can be seen as a horizontal band in the cervical body portion and a clear-grey vertical line extending from the incisal edge is evident. A small discoloured lesion is present at the centre of the CEJ (fig 209).

Upper right canine simulates the genetic condition amelogenesis imperfecta, a condition which prevents the enamel developing properly and causes extreme pitting on its surface.

Brown mauvish dentine colours are evident through the thin overlaying enamel at the incisal two-thirds of the tooth. A vertical discoloured crack is visible at the disto-labial corner.

All teeth have been fabricated to show the root formation at the CEJ (fig 210).

Palatal view illustrates dentine colour in the fossae and enamel marginal ridges.

Incisal translucency is evident demonstrating good light transmission from the labial side (fig 211).

10.2 Characteristic Details for Upper Anterior Porcelain Jacket Crowns

Aged Dentition

Maxillary central Duceram A3 displays many internal dentinal characteristics. Blue incisal border, yellow secondary dentine incisal third, internal brown stria, opalescent enamel at the mesial cervical corner, white enamel distal border reflects the underlying resin filling. Dentine halo effect is present due to the light scattering properties of the translucent enamel and the angle of the incisal edge.

Maxillary lateral in lighter shade. Duceram B2. Dentine mamelons are seen in the enamel. Translucent blue borders the incisal edge. Incisal edge profile displays typical wear pattern. Slight cleft at disto CEJ (fig 212).

Close detail distal aspect maxillary central illustrating worn resin filling (not used in clinical practice), and palatal view (figs 213 and 214).

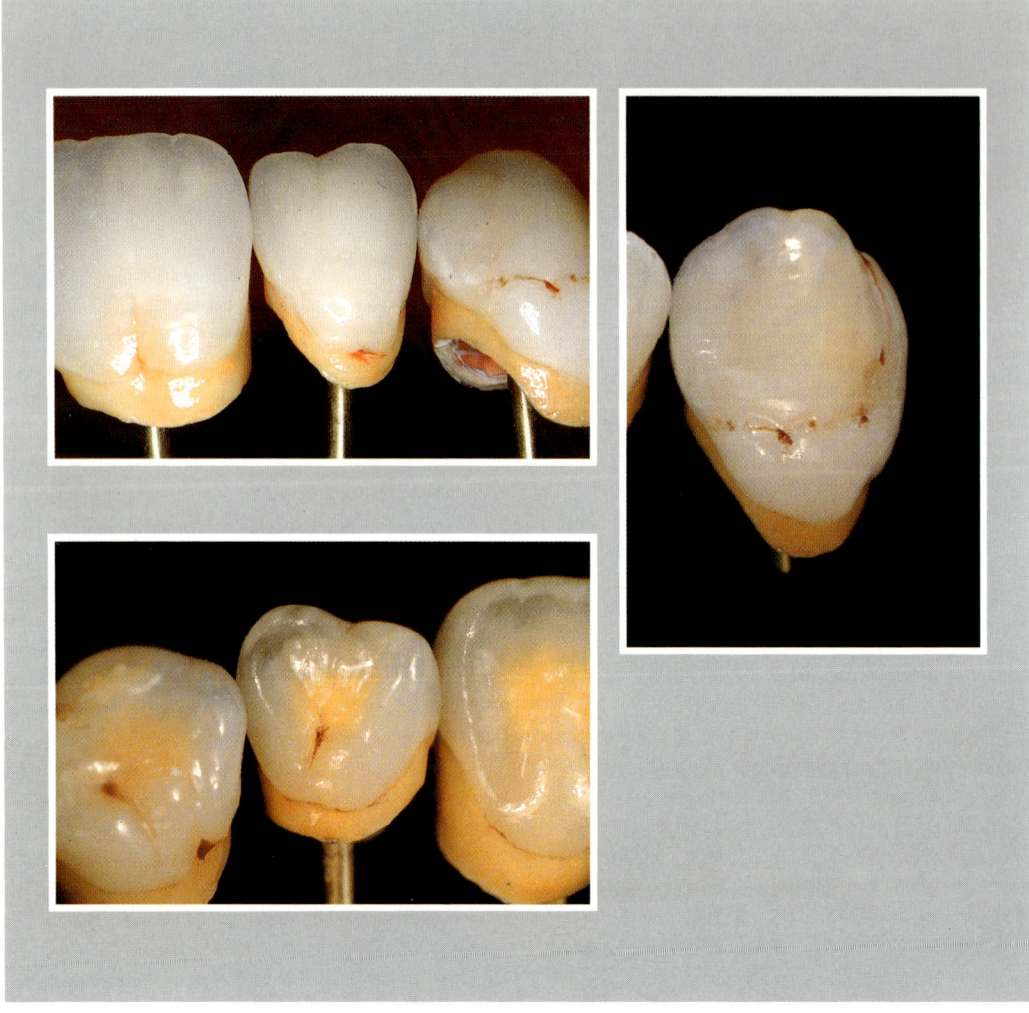

Phantom case depicts maxillary anterior teeth for the young dentition

Figs 209 to 211
Fig 209 (above left)   Typical mamelon characteristic and blue halo are present in the incisal area.

Fig 210 (right)   Maxillary canine simulates the abnormality Amelogenesis Imperfecta a condition which prevents the enamel forming correctly.

Fig 211 (below)   Palatal Aspect. Demonstrates depth of chroma in the fossae and white opalescent marginal ridges.

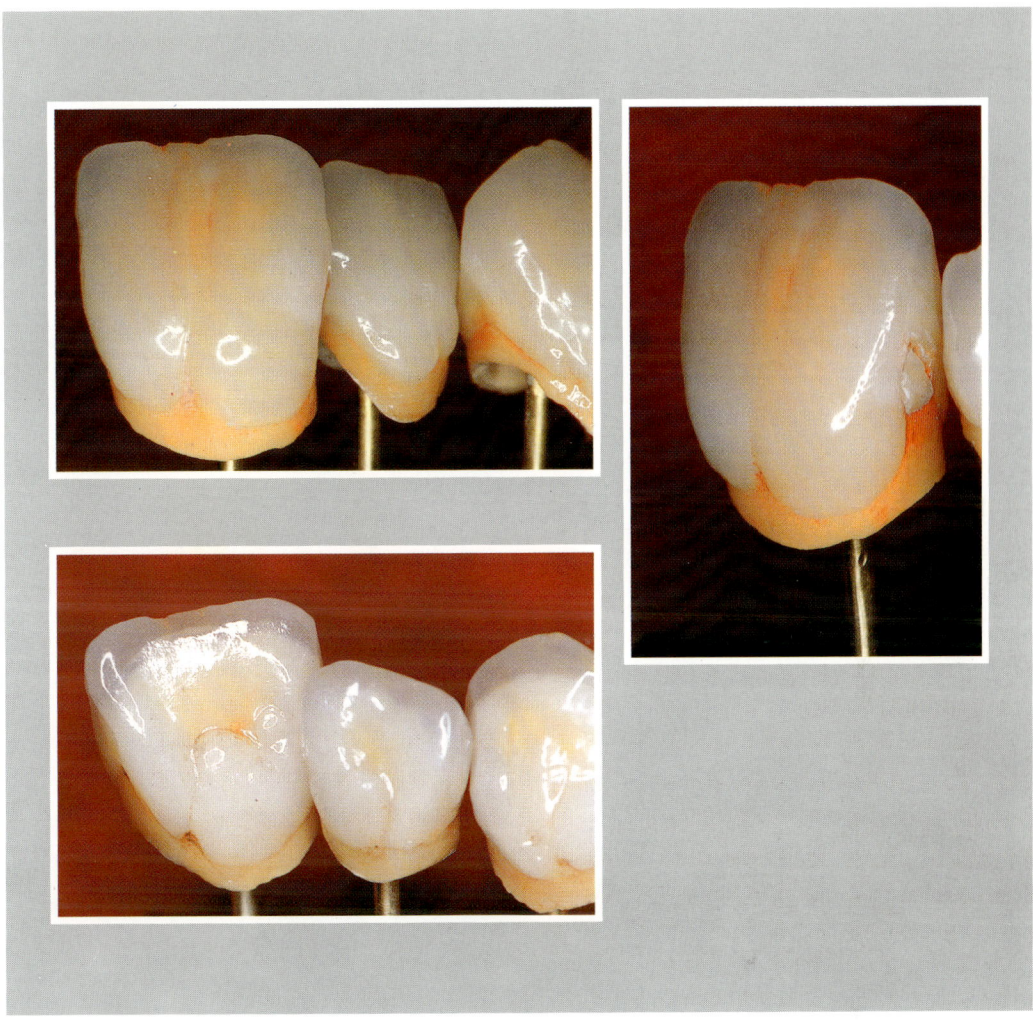

Phantom case depicts maxillary anterior teeth for the aged dentition

Figs 212 to 214
Fig 212 (above left)   Many internal colour characteristics are observed beneath the enamel. A worn composite filling is present at the distal wall of the central and a lighter area is visible on the facial aspect.

Fig 213 (right)   Close detail of the distal filling.

Fig 214 (below)   Palatal Aspect.

10.3 Characteristic Details for Mandibular Posterior Metal Ceramic Crowns

Posterior restorations for an elderly person

Individuality between teeth has been achieved by making use of different shades which will harmonise, in this case B4, C3, A4.

First Bicuspid
Yellow dentine colour is observed appearing through a thin translucent enamel overlay. White hyperplasia is present in the cervical region. Due to tissue recession the tooth root is exposed and a few discoloured pits are evident (fig 215).

Second Biscuspid
Facially the enamel layer is dense and whiter than the first bicuspid. A yellow tint is discernable in the occlusal third, as is a blue tint at the mesial development lobe. Opalescent enamel is present at the cervi-cal third and a brown crack extends from the CEJ towards the occlusal table on the distal side (figs 215 and 216).

The occlusal table is opalescent white with grey areas showing beneath the bucco-mesial marginal ridge and disto-lin-gual cusp tip (fig 217).

First molar
Facially this tooth has a horizontal band of tetracycline stain beneath a thin translucent enamel, a carious lesion at the mesial border is present and a second lesion is beginning between the cusp tips. Tissue reces-sion has exposed the root and a thin brown crack line appears between the cusps generating from the CEJ (figs 215 and 216).

Occlusal appearance. First and second bicuspid. Stained occlusal pits are evident. The second bicuspid mesio-lingual cusp displays an opalescent enamel. First molar illustrates central development fissure cari-ous lesion beneath the enamel.

Second lesion in the enamel is present at the bifurcation between mesial and distal cusp tips (fig 217).

Phantom case depicts aged dentition for the mandibular posterior teeth

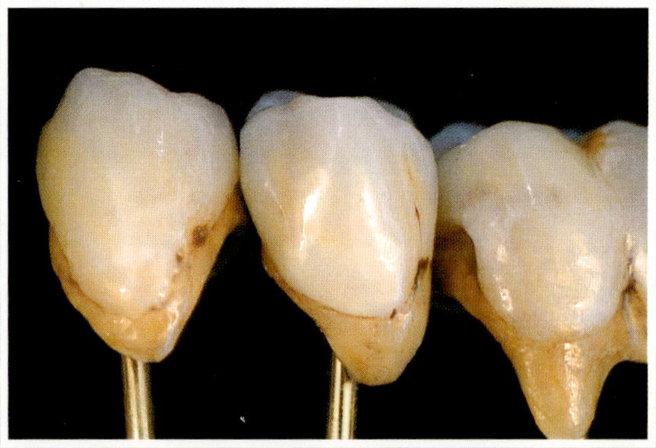

Figs 215 to 217
Fig 215 Depth of chroma, translucent opalescent enamel, root formation, internal characteristics together with crack lines, pits and enamel lesions are the many features of these teeth.

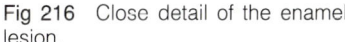

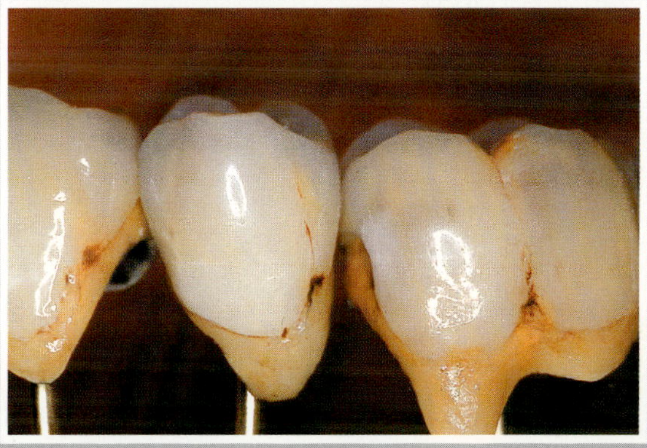

Fig 216 Close detail of the enamel lesion.

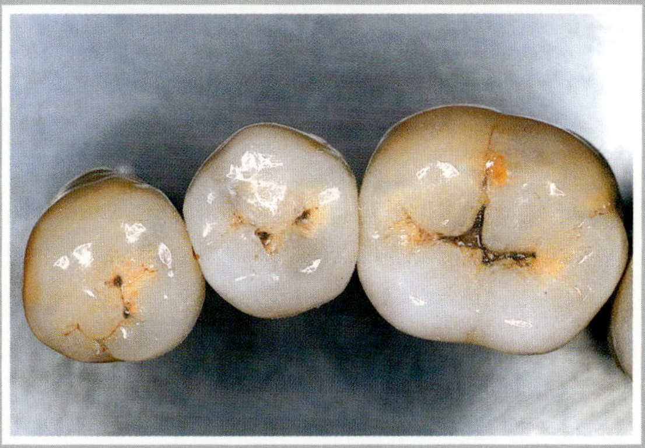

Fig 217 Occlusal view displays depth of chroma, surface pits and a lesion in the central fossae.

Phantom case constructed in 1983 fulfilling the requirements of the International Society for Dental Ceramics (ISDC) for fellowship status.

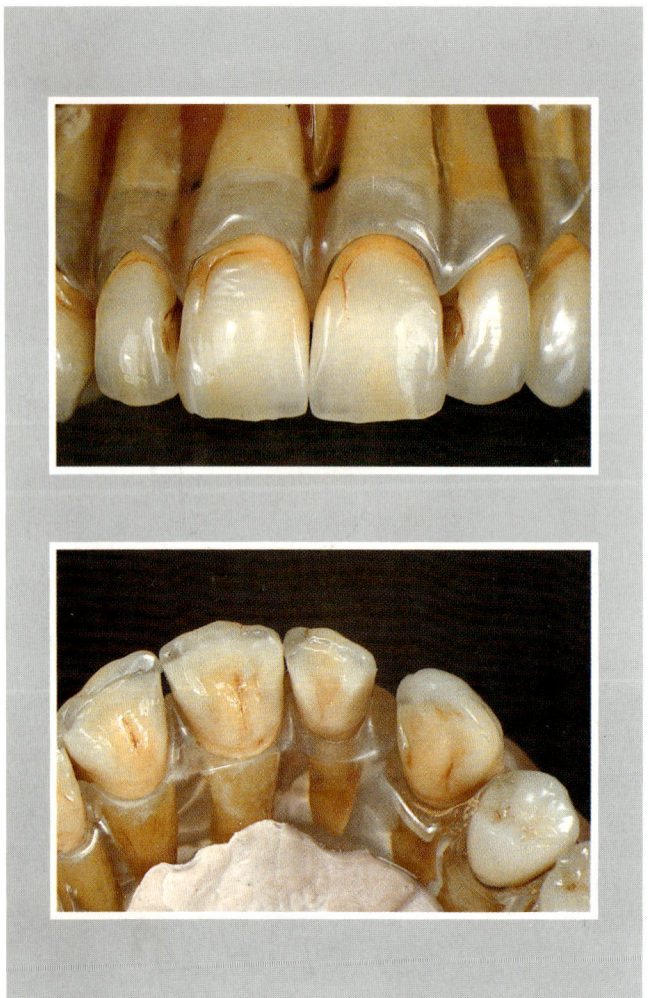

Fig 218 Anterior construction with 'Vitadur N' jacket crowns. A split post system was devised to allow inspection of the crown margins.

Fig 219 Palatal aspect. Note the use of high chroma dentine in the fossae and opalescent enamel on the marginal ridges.

Posterior construction

Figs 220 and 221
Good tooth morphology aids the aesthetic harmony of this case and high chroma dentines create individuality at the facial aspect as well as the illusion of depth in the occlusal fable.

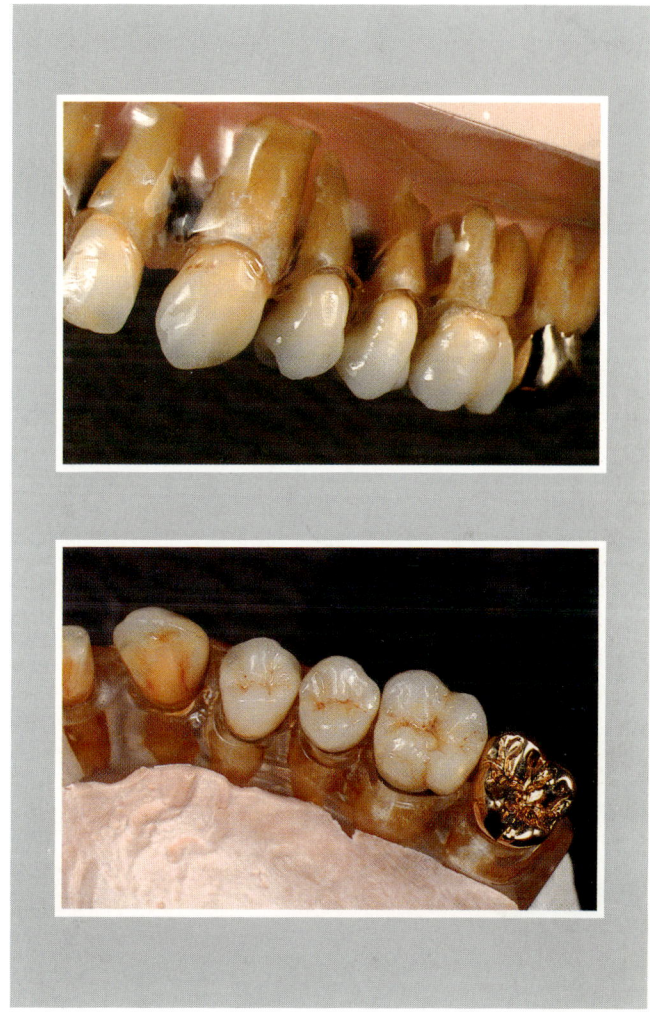